I0095403

THE BOOK BELONGS TO:

CONTACT INFORMATION	
NAME	
ADDRESS	
PHONE #	
EMAIL	

Copyright © Teresa Rother

All rights reserved. No part of this publication may be reproduced,
distributed, or transmitted in any form or by any means, including
photocopy, recording, or other electronic or mechanical methods.

BEFORE

AFTER

MEASUREMENTS	
DATE	
RIGHT ARM	
LEFT ARM	
WAIST	
HIPS	
RIGHT THIGH	
LEFT THIGH	
RIGHT CALF	
LEFT CALF	
BODY FAT%	
WEIGHT	

MEASUREMENTS	
DATE	
RIGHT ARM	
LEFT ARM	
WAIST	
HIPS	
RIGHT THIGH	
LEFT THIGH	
RIGHT CALF	
LEFT CALF	
BODY FAT%	
WEIGHT	

SHOPPING LIST

- O _____
- O _____
- O _____
- O _____
- O _____
- O _____
- O _____
- O _____
- O _____
- O _____
- O _____
- O _____
- O _____
- O _____
- O _____
- O _____
- O _____
- O _____
- O _____
- O _____
- O _____
- O _____
- O _____

- O _____
- O _____
- O _____
- O _____
- O _____
- O _____
- O _____
- O _____
- O _____
- O _____
- O _____
- O _____
- O _____
- O _____
- O _____
- O _____
- O _____
- O _____
- O _____
- O _____
- O _____
- O _____
- O _____

LOW CARB GROCERY LIST IDEAS

DAIRY

O Butter

O Cheese

O Cream Cheese

O Ghee

O Greek Yogurt, Full Fat

O Heavy Whipping Cream

O Mayo

O Sour Cream

O

O

O

O

O

O

O

O

O

O

O

O

O

O

O

PANTRY ITEMS

O Avocado Oil

O All-Natural Peanut Butter

O Almonds

O Almond Flour

O Almond Milk

O Beef Jerky

O Bone Broth

O Coconut Butter

O Coconut Oil

O Coffee/Tea

O Low Carb Protein Bars

O Low Carb Salad Dressing

O Mayonnaise

O Olive Oil, Extra Virgin

O Olives

O Pork Rinds

O Spices

O Stevia/Sweeteners

O Tuna/Salmon

O

O

O

O

O

O

LOW CARB GROCERY LIST IDEAS

FRESH PRODUCE

- O Asparagus
- O Avocados
- O Bell Peppers
- O Berries
- O Broccoli
- O Brussels Sprouts
- O Cabbage
- O Carrots
- O Cauliflower
- O Celery
- O Cucumber
- O Eggplant
- O Fennel
- O Garlic
- O Green Beans
- O Mushrooms
- O Onions
- O Radishes
- O Salad Mixes
- O Spinach
- O Squash
- O Tomatoes
- O
- O
- O

MEAT AND SEA FOOD

- O Bacon
- O Beef
- O Bison
- O Chicken
- O Deli Meat
- O Ground Beef
- O Ground Chicken
- O Lamb
- O Pork
- O Rotisserie Chicken
- O Sausage
- O Turkey
- O Fish
- O Crab
- O Lobster
- O Mussels
- O Oysters
- O Scallop
- O Shrimp
- O
- O
- O
- O
- O
- O

LOW CARB GROCERY LIST IDEAS

KETO FRIENDLY FOODS	NET CARBS	PROTEINS	FAT

KETOGENIC FOOD LIST

MEATS

Beef
Sausage
Bacon
Lamb
Pork
Veal
Chicken/Turkey
Eggs

VEGGIES

Avocado
Asparagus
Argula
Broccoli
Cauliflower
Brussel Sprouts
Cabbage
Celery

VEGGIES

Cucumber
Chards
Bell Peppers
Green Beans
Collards
Mushrooms
Spinach
Olives

FRUITS

Blackberries
Cranberries
Blueberries
Lemon
Lime
Raspberries
Strawberries
Plantains (paleo)

DAIRY

Cheese (all kinds)
Sour Cream
Cream Cheese
Heavy Cream
Greek Yogurt
Almond Milk
Cashew Milk
Coconut Cream

CONDIMENTS

Balsamic Vinegar
Beef/Chicken Broth
Bonito Flakes
Tartar Sauce (keto)
Dijon Mustard
Mayo
Low Sugar Ketchup
Pickles

OILS & FATS

Avocado Oil
Butter
Coconut Butter
Duck Fat
Lard/Ghee
Nut Oils
Olive Oil
Pork Rinds

HERBS & SPICES

Garlic
Salt & Pepper
Oregano
Paprika
Cumin
Chili Pepper
Basil
Ginger

BAKING

Almond Flour
Almond Meal
Cashew Flour
Oat Fiber
Psyllium Husk
Whey Protein
Flax meal
Hazelnut Flour

FISH/SEAFOOD

Anchovy
Haddock / Cod
Halibut
Crab/Lobster
Mackerel
Salmon
Tuna
Red Snapper

DRINKS

Diet Soda (moderation)
Coffee
Tea
Gatorade Zero
Protein Shake
Club Soda
Broth
Coconut Water

MISC.

Canned Tuna
Pesto
Soy Sauce
Aioli
Béarnaise
Vinaigrette
Hot Sauce
Guacamole

MACRO QUICK REFERENCE

MACRO TRACKER

QTY	TYPE	PROTEIN	FAT	CARBS	CALS	NOTES

MACRO QUICK REFERENCE

MACRO TRACKER

QTY	TYPE	PROTEIN	FAT	CARBS	CALS	NOTES

MACRO QUICK REFERENCE

MACRO TRACKER

QTY	TYPE	PROTEIN	FAT	CARBS	CALS	NOTES

DAILY TRACKER

DATE _____

SLEEP TRACKER:

☀ RISE: _____   🌙 zzz BEDTIME: _____   💤 zzz SLEEP (HRS): _____

EXERCISE			IN A STATE OF KETOSIS?		
TYPE	TIME	DURATION	YES	NO	UNSURE

CRAVINGS			DAILY ENERGY LEVEL		
YES	NO	SOMEWHAT	HIGH	MEDIUM	LOW

MEALS

	BREAKFAST	
	FAT	GRAMS
	CARBS	GRAMS
	PROTEIN	GRAMS
	CALORIES	

	LUNCH	
	FAT	GRAMS
	CARBS	GRAMS
	PROTEIN	GRAMS
	CALORIES	

	DINNER	
	FAT	GRAMS
	CARBS	GRAMS
	PROTEIN	GRAMS
	CALORIES	

	SNACK	
	FAT	GRAMS
	CARBS	GRAMS
	PROTEIN	GRAMS
	CALORIES	

	SNACK	
	FAT	GRAMS
	CARBS	GRAMS
	PROTEIN	GRAMS
	CALORIES	

WATER INTAKE TRACKER

💧 💧 💧 💧 💧 💧 💧 💧

END OF THE DAY TOTAL OVERVIEW

CARBS	FAT	PROTEIN	CALORIES

DAILY TRACKER

DATE _____

SLEEP TRACKER:

☀ RISE: [   ]   🌙 zzz BEDTIME: [   ]   💭 zzz SLEEP (HRS): [   ]

EXERCISE
TYPE   TIME   DURATION

IN A STATE OF KETOSIS?
YES   NO   UNSURE

CRAVINGS
YES   NO   SOMEWHAT

DAILY ENERGY LEVEL
HIGH   MEDIUM   LOW

MEALS

	BREAKFAST	
	FAT	GRAMS
	CARBS	GRAMS
	PROTEIN	GRAMS
	CALORIES	

	LUNCH	
	FAT	GRAMS
	CARBS	GRAMS
	PROTEIN	GRAMS
	CALORIES	

	DINNER	
	FAT	GRAMS
	CARBS	GRAMS
	PROTEIN	GRAMS
	CALORIES	

	SNACK	
	FAT	GRAMS
	CARBS	GRAMS
	PROTEIN	GRAMS
	CALORIES	

	SNACK	
	FAT	GRAMS
	CARBS	GRAMS
	PROTEIN	GRAMS
	CALORIES	

WATER INTAKE TRACKER

💧 💧 💧 💧 💧 💧 💧 💧

END OF THE DAY TOTAL OVERVIEW

CARBS	FAT	PROTEIN	CALORIES
[ ]	[ ]	[ ]	[ ]

DAILY TRACKER

DATE _____

SLEEP TRACKER:

☼ | RISE: | 🌙 zᶻ | BEDTIME: | 💭 zᶻᶻ | SLEEP (HRS):

EXERCISE			IN A STATE OF KETOSIS?		
TYPE	TIME	DURATION	YES	NO	UNSURE

CRAVINGS			DAILY ENERGY LEVEL		
YES	NO	SOMEWHAT	HIGH	MEDIUM	LOW

MEALS

BREAKFAST
FAT	GRAMS
CARBS	GRAMS
PROTEIN	GRAMS
CALORIES	

LUNCH
FAT	GRAMS
CARBS	GRAMS
PROTEIN	GRAMS
CALORIES	

DINNER
FAT	GRAMS
CARBS	GRAMS
PROTEIN	GRAMS
CALORIES	

SNACK
FAT	GRAMS
CARBS	GRAMS
PROTEIN	GRAMS
CALORIES	

SNACK
FAT	GRAMS
CARBS	GRAMS
PROTEIN	GRAMS
CALORIES	

WATER INTAKE TRACKER

💧 💧 💧 💧 💧 💧 💧 💧

END OF THE DAY TOTAL OVERVIEW

CARBS	FAT	PROTEIN	CALORIES

DAILY TRACKER

DATE _____

SLEEP TRACKER:

☼ RISE: | 🌙 BEDTIME: | 💭 SLEEP (HRS):

EXERCISE			IN A STATE OF KETOSIS?		
TYPE	TIME	DURATION	YES	NO	UNSURE

CRAVINGS			DAILY ENERGY LEVEL		
YES	NO	SOMEWHAT	HIGH	MEDIUM	LOW

MEALS

BREAKFAST
FAT	GRAMS
CARBS	GRAMS
PROTEIN	GRAMS
CALORIES	

LUNCH
FAT	GRAMS
CARBS	GRAMS
PROTEIN	GRAMS
CALORIES	

DINNER
FAT	GRAMS
CARBS	GRAMS
PROTEIN	GRAMS
CALORIES	

SNACK
FAT	GRAMS
CARBS	GRAMS
PROTEIN	GRAMS
CALORIES	

SNACK
FAT	GRAMS
CARBS	GRAMS
PROTEIN	GRAMS
CALORIES	

WATER INTAKE TRACKER

END OF THE DAY TOTAL OVERVIEW

CARBS	FAT	PROTEIN	CALORIES

DAILY TRACKER

DATE _____

SLEEP TRACKER:

☀ RISE: | 🌙 zzz BEDTIME: | 💤 SLEEP (HRS):

EXERCISE			IN A STATE OF KETOSIS?		
TYPE	TIME	DURATION	YES	NO	UNSURE

CRAVINGS			DAILY ENERGY LEVEL		
YES	NO	SOMEWHAT	HIGH	MEDIUM	LOW

MEALS

BREAKFAST
FAT · GRAMS
CARBS · GRAMS
PROTEIN · GRAMS
CALORIES

LUNCH
FAT · GRAMS
CARBS · GRAMS
PROTEIN · GRAMS
CALORIES

DINNER
FAT · GRAMS
CARBS · GRAMS
PROTEIN · GRAMS
CALORIES

SNACK
FAT · GRAMS
CARBS · GRAMS
PROTEIN · GRAMS
CALORIES

SNACK
FAT · GRAMS
CARBS · GRAMS
PROTEIN · GRAMS
CALORIES

WATER INTAKE TRACKER

END OF THE DAY TOTAL OVERVIEW

CARBS	FAT	PROTEIN	CALORIES

DAILY TRACKER

DATE _____

SLEEP TRACKER:

☀ RISE: [   ] 🌙 zzz BEDTIME: [   ] 💭 zzZ SLEEP (HRS): [   ]

EXERCISE			IN A STATE OF KETOSIS?		
TYPE	TIME	DURATION	YES	NO	UNSURE

CRAVINGS			DAILY ENERGY LEVEL		
YES	NO	SOMEWHAT	HIGH	MEDIUM	LOW

MEALS

	BREAKFAST	
	FAT	GRAMS
	CARBS	GRAMS
	PROTEIN	GRAMS
	CALORIES	
	LUNCH	
	FAT	GRAMS
	CARBS	GRAMS
	PROTEIN	GRAMS
	CALORIES	
	DINNER	
	FAT	GRAMS
	CARBS	GRAMS
	PROTEIN	GRAMS
	CALORIES	
	SNACK	
	FAT	GRAMS
	CARBS	GRAMS
	PROTEIN	GRAMS
	CALORIES	
	SNACK	
	FAT	GRAMS
	CARBS	GRAMS
	PROTEIN	GRAMS
	CALORIES	

WATER INTAKE TRACKER

💧 💧 💧 💧 💧 💧 💧 💧

END OF THE DAY TOTAL OVERVIEW

CARBS	FAT	PROTEIN	CALORIES
[ ]	[ ]	[ ]	[ ]

DAILY TRACKER

DATE _____

SLEEP TRACKER:

☼ RISE: _____   🌙 BEDTIME: _____   💤 SLEEP (HRS): _____

EXERCISE			IN A STATE OF KETOSIS?		
TYPE	TIME	DURATION	YES	NO	UNSURE

CRAVINGS			DAILY ENERGY LEVEL		
YES	NO	SOMEWHAT	HIGH	MEDIUM	LOW

MEALS

		BREAKFAST	
	FAT		GRAMS
	CARBS		GRAMS
	PROTEIN		GRAMS
	CALORIES		

		LUNCH	
	FAT		GRAMS
	CARBS		GRAMS
	PROTEIN		GRAMS
	CALORIES		

		DINNER	
	FAT		GRAMS
	CARBS		GRAMS
	PROTEIN		GRAMS
	CALORIES		

		SNACK	
	FAT		GRAMS
	CARBS		GRAMS
	PROTEIN		GRAMS
	CALORIES		

		SNACK	
	FAT		GRAMS
	CARBS		GRAMS
	PROTEIN		GRAMS
	CALORIES		

WATER INTAKE TRACKER

💧 💧 💧 💧 💧 💧 💧 💧

END OF THE DAY TOTAL OVERVIEW

CARBS	FAT	PROTEIN	CALORIES

DAILY TRACKER

DATE _____

SLEEP TRACKER:

☀ RISE: [ ] 🌙 BEDTIME: [ ] 💤 SLEEP (HRS): [ ]

EXERCISE			IN A STATE OF KETOSIS?		
TYPE	TIME	DURATION	YES	NO	UNSURE

CRAVINGS			DAILY ENERGY LEVEL		
YES	NO	SOMEWHAT	HIGH	MEDIUM	LOW

MEALS

	BREAKFAST
	FAT — GRAMS
	CARBS — GRAMS
	PROTEIN — GRAMS
	CALORIES
	LUNCH
	FAT — GRAMS
	CARBS — GRAMS
	PROTEIN — GRAMS
	CALORIES
	DINNER
	FAT — GRAMS
	CARBS — GRAMS
	PROTEIN — GRAMS
	CALORIES
	SNACK
	FAT — GRAMS
	CARBS — GRAMS
	PROTEIN — GRAMS
	CALORIES
	SNACK
	FAT — GRAMS
	CARBS — GRAMS
	PROTEIN — GRAMS
	CALORIES

WATER INTAKE TRACKER

💧 💧 💧 💧 💧 💧 💧 💧

END OF THE DAY TOTAL OVERVIEW

CARBS	FAT	PROTEIN	CALORIES
[ ]	[ ]	[ ]	[ ]

DAILY TRACKER

DATE _____

SLEEP TRACKER:

RISE: _____   BEDTIME: _____   SLEEP (HRS): _____

EXERCISE			IN A STATE OF KETOSIS?		
TYPE	TIME	DURATION	YES	NO	UNSURE

CRAVINGS			DAILY ENERGY LEVEL		
YES	NO	SOMEWHAT	HIGH	MEDIUM	LOW

MEALS

BREAKFAST

FAT	GRAMS
CARBS	GRAMS
PROTEIN	GRAMS
CALORIES	

LUNCH

FAT	GRAMS
CARBS	GRAMS
PROTEIN	GRAMS
CALORIES	

DINNER

FAT	GRAMS
CARBS	GRAMS
PROTEIN	GRAMS
CALORIES	

SNACK

FAT	GRAMS
CARBS	GRAMS
PROTEIN	GRAMS
CALORIES	

SNACK

FAT	GRAMS
CARBS	GRAMS
PROTEIN	GRAMS
CALORIES	

WATER INTAKE TRACKER

END OF THE DAY TOTAL OVERVIEW

CARBS	FAT	PROTEIN	CALORIES

DAILY TRACKER

DATE _____

SLEEP TRACKER:

☀ RISE: | 🌙 z z z BEDTIME: | 💤 z z z SLEEP (HRS):

EXERCISE			IN A STATE OF KETOSIS?		
TYPE	TIME	DURATION	YES	NO	UNSURE

CRAVINGS			DAILY ENERGY LEVEL		
YES	NO	SOMEWHAT	HIGH	MEDIUM	LOW

MEALS

	BREAKFAST	
	FAT	GRAMS
	CARBS	GRAMS
	PROTEIN	GRAMS
	CALORIES	

	LUNCH	
	FAT	GRAMS
	CARBS	GRAMS
	PROTEIN	GRAMS
	CALORIES	

	DINNER	
	FAT	GRAMS
	CARBS	GRAMS
	PROTEIN	GRAMS
	CALORIES	

	SNACK	
	FAT	GRAMS
	CARBS	GRAMS
	PROTEIN	GRAMS
	CALORIES	

	SNACK	
	FAT	GRAMS
	CARBS	GRAMS
	PROTEIN	GRAMS
	CALORIES	

WATER INTAKE TRACKER

END OF THE DAY TOTAL OVERVIEW

CARBS	FAT	PROTEIN	CALORIES

DAILY TRACKER

DATE _____

SLEEP TRACKER:

☀ | RISE: | 🌙 zzz | BEDTIME: | 💤 | SLEEP (HRS):

EXERCISE			IN A STATE OF KETOSIS?		
TYPE	TIME	DURATION	YES	NO	UNSURE

CRAVINGS			DAILY ENERGY LEVEL		
YES	NO	SOMEWHAT	HIGH	MEDIUM	LOW

MEALS

	BREAKFAST	
	FAT	GRAMS
	CARBS	GRAMS
	PROTEIN	GRAMS
	CALORIES	

	LUNCH	
	FAT	GRAMS
	CARBS	GRAMS
	PROTEIN	GRAMS
	CALORIES	

	DINNER	
	FAT	GRAMS
	CARBS	GRAMS
	PROTEIN	GRAMS
	CALORIES	

	SNACK	
	FAT	GRAMS
	CARBS	GRAMS
	PROTEIN	GRAMS
	CALORIES	

	SNACK	
	FAT	GRAMS
	CARBS	GRAMS
	PROTEIN	GRAMS
	CALORIES	

WATER INTAKE TRACKER

END OF THE DAY TOTAL OVERVIEW

CARBS	FAT	PROTEIN	CALORIES

DAILY TRACKER

DATE _____

SLEEP TRACKER:

☀ | RISE: | 🌙 z z z | BEDTIME: | 💤 | SLEEP (HRS):

EXERCISE			IN A STATE OF KETOSIS?		
TYPE	TIME	DURATION	YES	NO	UNSURE

CRAVINGS			DAILY ENERGY LEVEL		
YES	NO	SOMEWHAT	HIGH	MEDIUM	LOW

MEALS

BREAKFAST
FAT .... GRAMS
CARBS .... GRAMS
PROTEIN .... GRAMS
CALORIES

LUNCH
FAT .... GRAMS
CARBS .... GRAMS
PROTEIN .... GRAMS
CALORIES

DINNER
FAT .... GRAMS
CARBS .... GRAMS
PROTEIN .... GRAMS
CALORIES

SNACK
FAT .... GRAMS
CARBS .... GRAMS
PROTEIN .... GRAMS
CALORIES

SNACK
FAT .... GRAMS
CARBS .... GRAMS
PROTEIN .... GRAMS
CALORIES

WATER INTAKE TRACKER

END OF THE DAY TOTAL OVERVIEW

CARBS	FAT	PROTEIN	CALORIES

DAILY TRACKER

DATE _____

SLEEP TRACKER:

☀ RISE: _____ 🌙 zᶻz BEDTIME: _____ 💤 SLEEP (HRS): _____

EXERCISE			IN A STATE OF KETOSIS?		
TYPE	TIME	DURATION	YES	NO	UNSURE

CRAVINGS			DAILY ENERGY LEVEL		
YES	NO	SOMEWHAT	HIGH	MEDIUM	LOW

MEALS

BREAKFAST
FAT		GRAMS
CARBS		GRAMS
PROTEIN		GRAMS
CALORIES		

LUNCH
FAT		GRAMS
CARBS		GRAMS
PROTEIN		GRAMS
CALORIES		

DINNER
FAT		GRAMS
CARBS		GRAMS
PROTEIN		GRAMS
CALORIES		

SNACK
FAT		GRAMS
CARBS		GRAMS
PROTEIN		GRAMS
CALORIES		

SNACK
FAT		GRAMS
CARBS		GRAMS
PROTEIN		GRAMS
CALORIES		

WATER INTAKE TRACKER

END OF THE DAY TOTAL OVERVIEW

CARBS	FAT	PROTEIN	CALORIES

DAILY TRACKER

DATE _____

SLEEP TRACKER:

☀ RISE: _____   🌙 zᶻᶻ BEDTIME: _____   💭zᶻᶻ SLEEP (HRS): _____

EXERCISE			IN A STATE OF KETOSIS?		
TYPE	TIME	DURATION	YES	NO	UNSURE

CRAVINGS			DAILY ENERGY LEVEL		
YES	NO	SOMEWHAT	HIGH	MEDIUM	LOW

MEALS

	BREAKFAST	
	FAT	GRAMS
	CARBS	GRAMS
	PROTEIN	GRAMS
	CALORIES	

	LUNCH	
	FAT	GRAMS
	CARBS	GRAMS
	PROTEIN	GRAMS
	CALORIES	

	DINNER	
	FAT	GRAMS
	CARBS	GRAMS
	PROTEIN	GRAMS
	CALORIES	

	SNACK	
	FAT	GRAMS
	CARBS	GRAMS
	PROTEIN	GRAMS
	CALORIES	

	SNACK	
	FAT	GRAMS
	CARBS	GRAMS
	PROTEIN	GRAMS
	CALORIES	

WATER INTAKE TRACKER

END OF THE DAY TOTAL OVERVIEW

CARBS	FAT	PROTEIN	CALORIES

DAILY TRACKER

DATE _____

SLEEP TRACKER:

☀ RISE: _____   🌙 ᶻᶻᶻ BEDTIME: _____   💭ᶻᶻᶻ SLEEP (HRS): _____

EXERCISE			IN A STATE OF KETOSIS?		
TYPE	TIME	DURATION	YES	NO	UNSURE

CRAVINGS			DAILY ENERGY LEVEL		
YES	NO	SOMEWHAT	HIGH	MEDIUM	LOW

MEALS

	BREAKFAST	
	FAT	GRAMS
	CARBS	GRAMS
	PROTEIN	GRAMS
	CALORIES	

	LUNCH	
	FAT	GRAMS
	CARBS	GRAMS
	PROTEIN	GRAMS
	CALORIES	

	DINNER	
	FAT	GRAMS
	CARBS	GRAMS
	PROTEIN	GRAMS
	CALORIES	

	SNACK	
	FAT	GRAMS
	CARBS	GRAMS
	PROTEIN	GRAMS
	CALORIES	

	SNACK	
	FAT	GRAMS
	CARBS	GRAMS
	PROTEIN	GRAMS
	CALORIES	

WATER INTAKE TRACKER

END OF THE DAY TOTAL OVERVIEW

CARBS	FAT	PROTEIN	CALORIES

DAILY TRACKER

DATE _____

SLEEP TRACKER:

☀ RISE: _____   🌙 zᶻz BEDTIME: _____   💤 zᶻz SLEEP (HRS): _____

EXERCISE			IN A STATE OF KETOSIS?		
TYPE	TIME	DURATION	YES	NO	UNSURE

CRAVINGS			DAILY ENERGY LEVEL		
YES	NO	SOMEWHAT	HIGH	MEDIUM	LOW

MEALS

BREAKFAST
FAT	GRAMS
CARBS	GRAMS
PROTEIN	GRAMS
CALORIES	

LUNCH
FAT	GRAMS
CARBS	GRAMS
PROTEIN	GRAMS
CALORIES	

DINNER
FAT	GRAMS
CARBS	GRAMS
PROTEIN	GRAMS
CALORIES	

SNACK
FAT	GRAMS
CARBS	GRAMS
PROTEIN	GRAMS
CALORIES	

SNACK
FAT	GRAMS
CARBS	GRAMS
PROTEIN	GRAMS
CALORIES	

WATER INTAKE TRACKER

END OF THE DAY TOTAL OVERVIEW

CARBS	FAT	PROTEIN	CALORIES

DAILY TRACKER

DATE _____

SLEEP TRACKER:

☀ | RISE: _____ | 🌙 zᶻᶻ | BEDTIME: _____ | 💤 | SLEEP (HRS): _____

EXERCISE			IN A STATE OF KETOSIS?		
TYPE	TIME	DURATION	YES	NO	UNSURE

CRAVINGS			DAILY ENERGY LEVEL		
YES	NO	SOMEWHAT	HIGH	MEDIUM	LOW

MEALS

BREAKFAST
FAT .... GRAMS
CARBS .... GRAMS
PROTEIN .... GRAMS
CALORIES

LUNCH
FAT .... GRAMS
CARBS .... GRAMS
PROTEIN .... GRAMS
CALORIES

DINNER
FAT .... GRAMS
CARBS .... GRAMS
PROTEIN .... GRAMS
CALORIES

SNACK
FAT .... GRAMS
CARBS .... GRAMS
PROTEIN .... GRAMS
CALORIES

SNACK
FAT .... GRAMS
CARBS .... GRAMS
PROTEIN .... GRAMS
CALORIES

WATER INTAKE TRACKER

END OF THE DAY TOTAL OVERVIEW

CARBS	FAT	PROTEIN	CALORIES

DAILY TRACKER

DATE _____

SLEEP TRACKER:

☀ RISE: _____ 🌙 zᶻᶻ BEDTIME: _____ 💤 SLEEP (HRS): _____

EXERCISE			IN A STATE OF KETOSIS?		
TYPE	TIME	DURATION	YES	NO	UNSURE

CRAVINGS			DAILY ENERGY LEVEL		
YES	NO	SOMEWHAT	HIGH	MEDIUM	LOW

MEALS

BREAKFAST

FAT	GRAMS
CARBS	GRAMS
PROTEIN	GRAMS
CALORIES	

LUNCH

FAT	GRAMS
CARBS	GRAMS
PROTEIN	GRAMS
CALORIES	

DINNER

FAT	GRAMS
CARBS	GRAMS
PROTEIN	GRAMS
CALORIES	

SNACK

FAT	GRAMS
CARBS	GRAMS
PROTEIN	GRAMS
CALORIES	

SNACK

FAT	GRAMS
CARBS	GRAMS
PROTEIN	GRAMS
CALORIES	

WATER INTAKE TRACKER

💧 💧 💧 💧 💧 💧 💧 💧

END OF THE DAY TOTAL OVERVIEW

CARBS	FAT	PROTEIN	CALORIES

DAILY TRACKER

DATE _____

SLEEP TRACKER:

RISE: [_____]   BEDTIME: [_____]   SLEEP (HRS): [_____]

EXERCISE			IN A STATE OF KETOSIS?		
TYPE	TIME	DURATION	YES	NO	UNSURE

CRAVINGS			DAILY ENERGY LEVEL		
YES	NO	SOMEWHAT	HIGH	MEDIUM	LOW

MEALS

	BREAKFAST	
FAT		GRAMS
CARBS		GRAMS
PROTEIN		GRAMS
CALORIES		

	LUNCH	
FAT		GRAMS
CARBS		GRAMS
PROTEIN		GRAMS
CALORIES		

	DINNER	
FAT		GRAMS
CARBS		GRAMS
PROTEIN		GRAMS
CALORIES		

	SNACK	
FAT		GRAMS
CARBS		GRAMS
PROTEIN		GRAMS
CALORIES		

	SNACK	
FAT		GRAMS
CARBS		GRAMS
PROTEIN		GRAMS
CALORIES		

WATER INTAKE TRACKER

END OF THE DAY TOTAL OVERVIEW

CARBS	FAT	PROTEIN	CALORIES
[____]	[____]	[____]	[____]

DAILY TRACKER

DATE _____

SLEEP TRACKER:

☀ RISE: _____ 🌙 ᶻᶻᶻ BEDTIME: _____ 💤 SLEEP (HRS): _____

EXERCISE

TYPE   TIME   DURATION

IN A STATE OF KETOSIS?

YES   NO   UNSURE

CRAVINGS

YES   NO   SOMEWHAT

DAILY ENERGY LEVEL

HIGH   MEDIUM   LOW

MEALS

	BREAKFAST	
	FAT	GRAMS
	CARBS	GRAMS
	PROTEIN	GRAMS
	CALORIES	

	LUNCH	
	FAT	GRAMS
	CARBS	GRAMS
	PROTEIN	GRAMS
	CALORIES	

	DINNER	
	FAT	GRAMS
	CARBS	GRAMS
	PROTEIN	GRAMS
	CALORIES	

	SNACK	
	FAT	GRAMS
	CARBS	GRAMS
	PROTEIN	GRAMS
	CALORIES	

	SNACK	
	FAT	GRAMS
	CARBS	GRAMS
	PROTEIN	GRAMS
	CALORIES	

WATER INTAKE TRACKER

END OF THE DAY TOTAL OVERVIEW

CARBS   FAT   PROTEIN   CALORIES

DAILY TRACKER

DATE _____

SLEEP TRACKER:

☀ RISE: _____   🌙 zᶻz BEDTIME: _____   💭 zᶻZ SLEEP (HRS): _____

EXERCISE			IN A STATE OF KETOSIS?		
TYPE	TIME	DURATION	YES	NO	UNSURE

CRAVINGS			DAILY ENERGY LEVEL		
YES	NO	SOMEWHAT	HIGH	MEDIUM	LOW

MEALS

	BREAKFAST	
	FAT	GRAMS
	CARBS	GRAMS
	PROTEIN	GRAMS
	CALORIES	

	LUNCH	
	FAT	GRAMS
	CARBS	GRAMS
	PROTEIN	GRAMS
	CALORIES	

	DINNER	
	FAT	GRAMS
	CARBS	GRAMS
	PROTEIN	GRAMS
	CALORIES	

	SNACK	
	FAT	GRAMS
	CARBS	GRAMS
	PROTEIN	GRAMS
	CALORIES	

	SNACK	
	FAT	GRAMS
	CARBS	GRAMS
	PROTEIN	GRAMS
	CALORIES	

WATER INTAKE TRACKER

💧 💧 💧 💧 💧 💧 💧 💧

END OF THE DAY TOTAL OVERVIEW

CARBS	FAT	PROTEIN	CALORIES

DAILY TRACKER

DATE _____

SLEEP TRACKER:

☀ | RISE: _____ | 🌙 z z z | BEDTIME: _____ | 💤 | SLEEP (HRS): _____

EXERCISE

TYPE   TIME   DURATION

IN A STATE OF KETOSIS?

YES   NO   UNSURE

CRAVINGS

YES   NO   SOMEWHAT

DAILY ENERGY LEVEL

HIGH   MEDIUM   LOW

MEALS

BREAKFAST
FAT	GRAMS
CARBS	GRAMS
PROTEIN	GRAMS
CALORIES	

LUNCH
FAT	GRAMS
CARBS	GRAMS
PROTEIN	GRAMS
CALORIES	

DINNER
FAT	GRAMS
CARBS	GRAMS
PROTEIN	GRAMS
CALORIES	

SNACK
FAT	GRAMS
CARBS	GRAMS
PROTEIN	GRAMS
CALORIES	

SNACK
FAT	GRAMS
CARBS	GRAMS
PROTEIN	GRAMS
CALORIES	

WATER INTAKE TRACKER

💧 💧 💧 💧 💧 💧 💧 💧

END OF THE DAY TOTAL OVERVIEW

CARBS   FAT   PROTEIN   CALORIES

DAILY TRACKER

DATE _____

SLEEP TRACKER:

☼ | RISE: | 🌙 zzᶻ | BEDTIME: | 💤 | SLEEP (HRS): |

EXERCISE			IN A STATE OF KETOSIS?		
TYPE	TIME	DURATION	YES	NO	UNSURE

CRAVINGS			DAILY ENERGY LEVEL		
YES	NO	SOMEWHAT	HIGH	MEDIUM	LOW

MEALS

BREAKFAST
FAT	GRAMS
CARBS	GRAMS
PROTEIN	GRAMS
CALORIES	

LUNCH
FAT	GRAMS
CARBS	GRAMS
PROTEIN	GRAMS
CALORIES	

DINNER
FAT	GRAMS
CARBS	GRAMS
PROTEIN	GRAMS
CALORIES	

SNACK
FAT	GRAMS
CARBS	GRAMS
PROTEIN	GRAMS
CALORIES	

SNACK
FAT	GRAMS
CARBS	GRAMS
PROTEIN	GRAMS
CALORIES	

WATER INTAKE TRACKER

END OF THE DAY TOTAL OVERVIEW

CARBS	FAT	PROTEIN	CALORIES

DAILY TRACKER

DATE _____

SLEEP TRACKER:

☀ RISE: _____   🌙 BEDTIME: _____   💤 SLEEP (HRS): _____

EXERCISE

TYPE   TIME   DURATION

IN A STATE OF KETOSIS?

YES   NO   UNSURE

CRAVINGS

YES   NO   SOMEWHAT

DAILY ENERGY LEVEL

HIGH   MEDIUM   LOW

MEALS

	BREAKFAST	
	FAT	GRAMS
	CARBS	GRAMS
	PROTEIN	GRAMS
	CALORIES	

	LUNCH	
	FAT	GRAMS
	CARBS	GRAMS
	PROTEIN	GRAMS
	CALORIES	

	DINNER	
	FAT	GRAMS
	CARBS	GRAMS
	PROTEIN	GRAMS
	CALORIES	

	SNACK	
	FAT	GRAMS
	CARBS	GRAMS
	PROTEIN	GRAMS
	CALORIES	

	SNACK	
	FAT	GRAMS
	CARBS	GRAMS
	PROTEIN	GRAMS
	CALORIES	

WATER INTAKE TRACKER

END OF THE DAY TOTAL OVERVIEW

CARBS   FAT   PROTEIN   CALORIES

DAILY TRACKER

DATE _____

SLEEP TRACKER:

RISE: _____   BEDTIME: _____   SLEEP (HRS): _____

EXERCISE			IN A STATE OF KETOSIS?		
TYPE	TIME	DURATION	YES	NO	UNSURE

CRAVINGS			DAILY ENERGY LEVEL		
YES	NO	SOMEWHAT	HIGH	MEDIUM	LOW

MEALS

	BREAKFAST	
	FAT	GRAMS
	CARBS	GRAMS
	PROTEIN	GRAMS
	CALORIES	

	LUNCH	
	FAT	GRAMS
	CARBS	GRAMS
	PROTEIN	GRAMS
	CALORIES	

	DINNER	
	FAT	GRAMS
	CARBS	GRAMS
	PROTEIN	GRAMS
	CALORIES	

	SNACK	
	FAT	GRAMS
	CARBS	GRAMS
	PROTEIN	GRAMS
	CALORIES	

	SNACK	
	FAT	GRAMS
	CARBS	GRAMS
	PROTEIN	GRAMS
	CALORIES	

WATER INTAKE TRACKER

END OF THE DAY TOTAL OVERVIEW

CARBS	FAT	PROTEIN	CALORIES

DAILY TRACKER

DATE _____

SLEEP TRACKER:

☼ | RISE: | 🌙 zᶻᶻ | BEDTIME: | 💭 zᶻᶻ | SLEEP (HRS):

EXERCISE			IN A STATE OF KETOSIS?		
TYPE	TIME	DURATION	YES	NO	UNSURE

CRAVINGS			DAILY ENERGY LEVEL		
YES	NO	SOMEWHAT	HIGH	MEDIUM	LOW

MEALS

BREAKFAST
FAT	GRAMS
CARBS	GRAMS
PROTEIN	GRAMS
CALORIES	

LUNCH
FAT	GRAMS
CARBS	GRAMS
PROTEIN	GRAMS
CALORIES	

DINNER
FAT	GRAMS
CARBS	GRAMS
PROTEIN	GRAMS
CALORIES	

SNACK
FAT	GRAMS
CARBS	GRAMS
PROTEIN	GRAMS
CALORIES	

SNACK
FAT	GRAMS
CARBS	GRAMS
PROTEIN	GRAMS
CALORIES	

WATER INTAKE TRACKER

END OF THE DAY TOTAL OVERVIEW

CARBS	FAT	PROTEIN	CALORIES

DAILY TRACKER

DATE _____

SLEEP TRACKER:

☼ RISE:	🌙 BEDTIME:	💤 SLEEP (HRS):

EXERCISE

TYPE	TIME	DURATION

IN A STATE OF KETOSIS?

YES   NO   UNSURE

CRAVINGS

YES   NO   SOMEWHAT

DAILY ENERGY LEVEL

HIGH   MEDIUM   LOW

MEALS

	BREAKFAST	
	FAT	GRAMS
	CARBS	GRAMS
	PROTEIN	GRAMS
	CALORIES	

	LUNCH	
	FAT	GRAMS
	CARBS	GRAMS
	PROTEIN	GRAMS
	CALORIES	

	DINNER	
	FAT	GRAMS
	CARBS	GRAMS
	PROTEIN	GRAMS
	CALORIES	

	SNACK	
	FAT	GRAMS
	CARBS	GRAMS
	PROTEIN	GRAMS
	CALORIES	

	SNACK	
	FAT	GRAMS
	CARBS	GRAMS
	PROTEIN	GRAMS
	CALORIES	

WATER INTAKE TRACKER

END OF THE DAY TOTAL OVERVIEW

CARBS	FAT	PROTEIN	CALORIES

DAILY TRACKER

DATE _____

SLEEP TRACKER:

☀ RISE: _____   🌙 zᶻᶻ BEDTIME: _____   💤 zᶻᶻ SLEEP (HRS): _____

EXERCISE			IN A STATE OF KETOSIS?		
TYPE	TIME	DURATION	YES	NO	UNSURE

CRAVINGS			DAILY ENERGY LEVEL		
YES	NO	SOMEWHAT	HIGH	MEDIUM	LOW

MEALS

BREAKFAST

FAT	GRAMS
CARBS	GRAMS
PROTEIN	GRAMS
CALORIES	

LUNCH

FAT	GRAMS
CARBS	GRAMS
PROTEIN	GRAMS
CALORIES	

DINNER

FAT	GRAMS
CARBS	GRAMS
PROTEIN	GRAMS
CALORIES	

SNACK

FAT	GRAMS
CARBS	GRAMS
PROTEIN	GRAMS
CALORIES	

SNACK

FAT	GRAMS
CARBS	GRAMS
PROTEIN	GRAMS
CALORIES	

WATER INTAKE TRACKER

END OF THE DAY TOTAL OVERVIEW

CARBS	FAT	PROTEIN	CALORIES

DAILY TRACKER

DATE _____

SLEEP TRACKER:

☀ RISE: [   ]   ☾ᶻᶻᶻ BEDTIME: [   ]   💤 SLEEP (HRS): [   ]

EXERCISE			IN A STATE OF KETOSIS?		
TYPE	TIME	DURATION	YES	NO	UNSURE

CRAVINGS			DAILY ENERGY LEVEL		
YES	NO	SOMEWHAT	HIGH	MEDIUM	LOW

MEALS

	BREAKFAST	
	FAT	GRAMS
	CARBS	GRAMS
	PROTEIN	GRAMS
	CALORIES	

	LUNCH	
	FAT	GRAMS
	CARBS	GRAMS
	PROTEIN	GRAMS
	CALORIES	

	DINNER	
	FAT	GRAMS
	CARBS	GRAMS
	PROTEIN	GRAMS
	CALORIES	

	SNACK	
	FAT	GRAMS
	CARBS	GRAMS
	PROTEIN	GRAMS
	CALORIES	

	SNACK	
	FAT	GRAMS
	CARBS	GRAMS
	PROTEIN	GRAMS
	CALORIES	

WATER INTAKE TRACKER

💧 💧 💧 💧 💧 💧 💧 💧

END OF THE DAY TOTAL OVERVIEW

CARBS	FAT	PROTEIN	CALORIES
[ ]	[ ]	[ ]	[ ]

DAILY TRACKER

DATE _____

SLEEP TRACKER:

☀ RISE: _____ 🌙 zᶻᶻ BEDTIME: _____ 💤 SLEEP (HRS): _____

EXERCISE			IN A STATE OF KETOSIS?		
TYPE	TIME	DURATION	YES	NO	UNSURE

CRAVINGS			DAILY ENERGY LEVEL		
YES	NO	SOMEWHAT	HIGH	MEDIUM	LOW

MEALS

	BREAKFAST	
FAT		GRAMS
CARBS		GRAMS
PROTEIN		GRAMS
CALORIES		

	LUNCH	
FAT		GRAMS
CARBS		GRAMS
PROTEIN		GRAMS
CALORIES		

	DINNER	
FAT		GRAMS
CARBS		GRAMS
PROTEIN		GRAMS
CALORIES		

	SNACK	
FAT		GRAMS
CARBS		GRAMS
PROTEIN		GRAMS
CALORIES		

	SNACK	
FAT		GRAMS
CARBS		GRAMS
PROTEIN		GRAMS
CALORIES		

WATER INTAKE TRACKER

END OF THE DAY TOTAL OVERVIEW

CARBS	FAT	PROTEIN	CALORIES

INTERMITTENT FASTING

DATES:			
	START TIME	END TIME	TOTAL HOURS
MON			
TUE	:	:	
WED	:	:	
THU	;	;	
FRI	:	:	
SAT	:	:	
SUN	:	:	

DATES:			
	START TIME	END TIME	TOTAL HOURS
MON			
TUE	:	:	
WED	:	:	
THU	;	;	
FRI	:	:	
SAT	:	:	
SUN	:	:	

DATES:			
	START TIME	END TIME	TOTAL HOURS
MON			
TUE	:	:	
WED	:	:	
THU	;	;	
FRI	:	:	
SAT	:	:	
SUN	:	:	

DATES:			
	START TIME	END TIME	TOTAL HOURS
MON			
TUE	:	:	
WED	:	:	
THU	;	;	
FRI	:	:	
SAT	:	:	
SUN	:	:	

DATES:			
	START TIME	END TIME	TOTAL HOURS
MON			
TUE	:	:	
WED	:	:	
THU	;	;	
FRI	:	:	
SAT	:	:	
SUN	:	:	

DATES:			
	START TIME	END TIME	TOTAL HOURS
MON			
TUE	:	:	
WED	:	:	
THU	;	;	
FRI	:	:	
SAT	:	:	
SUN	:	:	

DATES:			
	START TIME	END TIME	TOTAL HOURS
MON			
TUE	:	:	
WED	:	:	
THU	;	;	
FRI	:	:	
SAT	:	:	
SUN	:	:	

DATES:			
	START TIME	END TIME	TOTAL HOURS
MON			
TUE	:	:	
WED	:	:	
THU	;	;	
FRI	:	:	
SAT	:	:	
SUN	:	:	

DATES:			
	START TIME	END TIME	TOTAL HOURS
MON			
TUE	:	:	
WED	:	:	
THU	;	;	
FRI	:	:	
SAT	:	:	
SUN	:	:	

NOTES

INTERMITTENT FASTING

DATES:

	START TIME	END TIME	TOTAL HOURS
MON			
TUE	:	:	
WED	:	:	
THU	;	;	
FRI	:	:	
SAT	:	:	
SUN	:	:	

DATES:

	START TIME	END TIME	TOTAL HOURS
MON			
TUE	:	:	
WED	:	:	
THU	;	;	
FRI	:	:	
SAT	:	:	
SUN	:	:	

DATES:

	START TIME	END TIME	TOTAL HOURS
MON			
TUE	:	:	
WED	:	:	
THU	;	;	
FRI	:	:	
SAT	:	:	
SUN	:	:	

DATES:

	START TIME	END TIME	TOTAL HOURS
MON			
TUE	:	:	
WED	:	:	
THU	;	;	
FRI	:	:	
SAT	:	:	
SUN	:	:	

DATES:

	START TIME	END TIME	TOTAL HOURS
MON			
TUE	:	:	
WED	:	:	
THU	;	;	
FRI	:	:	
SAT	:	:	
SUN	:	:	

DATES:

	START TIME	END TIME	TOTAL HOURS
MON			
TUE	:	:	
WED	:	:	
THU	;	;	
FRI	:	:	
SAT	:	:	
SUN	:	:	

DATES:

	START TIME	END TIME	TOTAL HOURS
MON			
TUE	:	:	
WED	:	:	
THU	;	;	
FRI	:	:	
SAT	:	:	
SUN	:	:	

DATES:

	START TIME	END TIME	TOTAL HOURS
MON			
TUE	:	:	
WED	:	:	
THU	;	;	
FRI	:	:	
SAT	:	:	
SUN	:	:	

DATES:

	START TIME	END TIME	TOTAL HOURS
MON			
TUE	:	:	
WED	:	:	
THU	;	;	
FRI	:	:	
SAT	:	:	
SUN	:	:	

NOTES

30 DAYS OF KETO

STARTING WEIGHT:

DAY 30 WEIGHT:

(1) (2) (3) (4) (5) (6) (7) (8) (9) (10)

LBS LOST:

INCHES LOST:

(11) (12) (13) (14) (15) (16) (17) (18) (19) (20)

LBS LOST:

INCHES LOST:

(21) (22) (23) (24) (25) (26) (27) (28) (29) (30)

LBS LOST:

INCHES LOST:

TOTAL WEIGHT LOST:

TOTAL INCHES LOST:

THOUGHTS & REFLECTIONS:

DAILY TRACKER

DATE _____

SLEEP TRACKER:

RISE: _____   BEDTIME: _____   SLEEP (HRS): _____

EXERCISE			IN A STATE OF KETOSIS?		
TYPE	TIME	DURATION	YES	NO	UNSURE

CRAVINGS			DAILY ENERGY LEVEL		
YES	NO	SOMEWHAT	HIGH	MEDIUM	LOW

MEALS

BREAKFAST
FAT	GRAMS
CARBS	GRAMS
PROTEIN	GRAMS
CALORIES	

LUNCH
FAT	GRAMS
CARBS	GRAMS
PROTEIN	GRAMS
CALORIES	

DINNER
FAT	GRAMS
CARBS	GRAMS
PROTEIN	GRAMS
CALORIES	

SNACK
FAT	GRAMS
CARBS	GRAMS
PROTEIN	GRAMS
CALORIES	

SNACK
FAT	GRAMS
CARBS	GRAMS
PROTEIN	GRAMS
CALORIES	

WATER INTAKE TRACKER

END OF THE DAY TOTAL OVERVIEW

CARBS	FAT	PROTEIN	CALORIES

DAILY TRACKER

DATE _____

SLEEP TRACKER:

☀ | RISE: | 🌙 | BEDTIME: | 💤 | SLEEP (HRS):

EXERCISE			IN A STATE OF KETOSIS?		
TYPE	TIME	DURATION	YES	NO	UNSURE

CRAVINGS			DAILY ENERGY LEVEL		
YES	NO	SOMEWHAT	HIGH	MEDIUM	LOW

MEALS

	BREAKFAST	
	FAT	GRAMS
	CARBS	GRAMS
	PROTEIN	GRAMS
	CALORIES	

	LUNCH	
	FAT	GRAMS
	CARBS	GRAMS
	PROTEIN	GRAMS
	CALORIES	

	DINNER	
	FAT	GRAMS
	CARBS	GRAMS
	PROTEIN	GRAMS
	CALORIES	

	SNACK	
	FAT	GRAMS
	CARBS	GRAMS
	PROTEIN	GRAMS
	CALORIES	

	SNACK	
	FAT	GRAMS
	CARBS	GRAMS
	PROTEIN	GRAMS
	CALORIES	

WATER INTAKE TRACKER

💧 💧 💧 💧 💧 💧 💧 💧

END OF THE DAY TOTAL OVERVIEW

CARBS	FAT	PROTEIN	CALORIES

DAILY TRACKER

DATE _____

SLEEP TRACKER:

☀ RISE: [   ]   🌙 ᶻᶻᶻ BEDTIME: [   ]   💭 ᶻᶻᶻ SLEEP (HRS): [   ]

EXERCISE			IN A STATE OF KETOSIS?		
TYPE	TIME	DURATION	YES	NO	UNSURE

CRAVINGS			DAILY ENERGY LEVEL		
YES	NO	SOMEWHAT	HIGH	MEDIUM	LOW

MEALS

	BREAKFAST	
	FAT	GRAMS
	CARBS	GRAMS
	PROTEIN	GRAMS
	CALORIES	

	LUNCH	
	FAT	GRAMS
	CARBS	GRAMS
	PROTEIN	GRAMS
	CALORIES	

	DINNER	
	FAT	GRAMS
	CARBS	GRAMS
	PROTEIN	GRAMS
	CALORIES	

	SNACK	
	FAT	GRAMS
	CARBS	GRAMS
	PROTEIN	GRAMS
	CALORIES	

	SNACK	
	FAT	GRAMS
	CARBS	GRAMS
	PROTEIN	GRAMS
	CALORIES	

WATER INTAKE TRACKER

💧 💧 💧 💧 💧 💧 💧 💧

END OF THE DAY TOTAL OVERVIEW

CARBS	FAT	PROTEIN	CALORIES
[ ]	[ ]	[ ]	[ ]

DAILY TRACKER

DATE _____

SLEEP TRACKER:

☀ RISE: _____   🌙 ᶻᶻᶻ BEDTIME: _____   💭 ᶻᶻᶻ SLEEP (HRS): _____

EXERCISE			IN A STATE OF KETOSIS?		
TYPE	TIME	DURATION	YES	NO	UNSURE

CRAVINGS			DAILY ENERGY LEVEL		
YES	NO	SOMEWHAT	HIGH	MEDIUM	LOW

MEALS

	BREAKFAST	
	FAT	GRAMS
	CARBS	GRAMS
	PROTEIN	GRAMS
	CALORIES	

	LUNCH	
	FAT	GRAMS
	CARBS	GRAMS
	PROTEIN	GRAMS
	CALORIES	

	DINNER	
	FAT	GRAMS
	CARBS	GRAMS
	PROTEIN	GRAMS
	CALORIES	

	SNACK	
	FAT	GRAMS
	CARBS	GRAMS
	PROTEIN	GRAMS
	CALORIES	

	SNACK	
	FAT	GRAMS
	CARBS	GRAMS
	PROTEIN	GRAMS
	CALORIES	

WATER INTAKE TRACKER

💧 💧 💧 💧 💧 💧 💧 💧

END OF THE DAY TOTAL OVERVIEW

CARBS	FAT	PROTEIN	CALORIES

DAILY TRACKER

DATE _____

SLEEP TRACKER:

RISE: _____   BEDTIME: _____   SLEEP (HRS): _____

EXERCISE				IN A STATE OF KETOSIS?		
TYPE	TIME	DURATION		YES	NO	UNSURE

CRAVINGS				DAILY ENERGY LEVEL		
YES	NO	SOMEWHAT		HIGH	MEDIUM	LOW

MEALS

	BREAKFAST
	FAT .... GRAMS
	CARBS .... GRAMS
	PROTEIN .... GRAMS
	CALORIES

	LUNCH
	FAT .... GRAMS
	CARBS .... GRAMS
	PROTEIN .... GRAMS
	CALORIES

	DINNER
	FAT .... GRAMS
	CARBS .... GRAMS
	PROTEIN .... GRAMS
	CALORIES

	SNACK
	FAT .... GRAMS
	CARBS .... GRAMS
	PROTEIN .... GRAMS
	CALORIES

	SNACK
	FAT .... GRAMS
	CARBS .... GRAMS
	PROTEIN .... GRAMS
	CALORIES

WATER INTAKE TRACKER

END OF THE DAY TOTAL OVERVIEW

CARBS	FAT	PROTEIN	CALORIES

DAILY TRACKER

DATE _____

SLEEP TRACKER:

☀ RISE: 🌙 BEDTIME: 💭 SLEEP (HRS):

EXERCISE			IN A STATE OF KETOSIS?		
TYPE	TIME	DURATION	YES	NO	UNSURE

CRAVINGS			DAILY ENERGY LEVEL		
YES	NO	SOMEWHAT	HIGH	MEDIUM	LOW

MEALS

	BREAKFAST	
	FAT	GRAMS
	CARBS	GRAMS
	PROTEIN	GRAMS
	CALORIES	

	LUNCH	
	FAT	GRAMS
	CARBS	GRAMS
	PROTEIN	GRAMS
	CALORIES	

	DINNER	
	FAT	GRAMS
	CARBS	GRAMS
	PROTEIN	GRAMS
	CALORIES	

	SNACK	
	FAT	GRAMS
	CARBS	GRAMS
	PROTEIN	GRAMS
	CALORIES	

	SNACK	
	FAT	GRAMS
	CARBS	GRAMS
	PROTEIN	GRAMS
	CALORIES	

WATER INTAKE TRACKER

END OF THE DAY TOTAL OVERVIEW

CARBS	FAT	PROTEIN	CALORIES

DAILY TRACKER

DATE _____

SLEEP TRACKER:

☼ RISE: _____   🌙 zᶻᶻ BEDTIME: _____   💭zᶻᶻ SLEEP (HRS): _____

EXERCISE			IN A STATE OF KETOSIS?		
TYPE	TIME	DURATION	YES	NO	UNSURE

CRAVINGS			DAILY ENERGY LEVEL		
YES	NO	SOMEWHAT	HIGH	MEDIUM	LOW

MEALS

	BREAKFAST	
	FAT	GRAMS
	CARBS	GRAMS
	PROTEIN	GRAMS
	CALORIES	

	LUNCH	
	FAT	GRAMS
	CARBS	GRAMS
	PROTEIN	GRAMS
	CALORIES	

	DINNER	
	FAT	GRAMS
	CARBS	GRAMS
	PROTEIN	GRAMS
	CALORIES	

	SNACK	
	FAT	GRAMS
	CARBS	GRAMS
	PROTEIN	GRAMS
	CALORIES	

	SNACK	
	FAT	GRAMS
	CARBS	GRAMS
	PROTEIN	GRAMS
	CALORIES	

WATER INTAKE TRACKER

END OF THE DAY TOTAL OVERVIEW

CARBS	FAT	PROTEIN	CALORIES

DAILY TRACKER

DATE _____

SLEEP TRACKER:

☀ RISE: _____   🌙 z z z BEDTIME: _____   💤 z z z SLEEP (HRS): _____

EXERCISE			IN A STATE OF KETOSIS?		
TYPE	TIME	DURATION	YES	NO	UNSURE

CRAVINGS			DAILY ENERGY LEVEL		
YES	NO	SOMEWHAT	HIGH	MEDIUM	LOW

MEALS

BREAKFAST

FAT	GRAMS
CARBS	GRAMS
PROTEIN	GRAMS
CALORIES	

LUNCH

FAT	GRAMS
CARBS	GRAMS
PROTEIN	GRAMS
CALORIES	

DINNER

FAT	GRAMS
CARBS	GRAMS
PROTEIN	GRAMS
CALORIES	

SNACK

FAT	GRAMS
CARBS	GRAMS
PROTEIN	GRAMS
CALORIES	

SNACK

FAT	GRAMS
CARBS	GRAMS
PROTEIN	GRAMS
CALORIES	

WATER INTAKE TRACKER

END OF THE DAY TOTAL OVERVIEW

CARBS	FAT	PROTEIN	CALORIES

DAILY TRACKER

DATE _____

SLEEP TRACKER:

☼ | RISE: | 🌙 zᶻᶻ | BEDTIME: | 💭zᶻᶻ | SLEEP (HRS):

EXERCISE			IN A STATE OF KETOSIS?		
TYPE	TIME	DURATION	YES	NO	UNSURE

CRAVINGS			DAILY ENERGY LEVEL		
YES	NO	SOMEWHAT	HIGH	MEDIUM	LOW

MEALS

BREAKFAST
FAT	GRAMS
CARBS	GRAMS
PROTEIN	GRAMS
CALORIES	

LUNCH
FAT	GRAMS
CARBS	GRAMS
PROTEIN	GRAMS
CALORIES	

DINNER
FAT	GRAMS
CARBS	GRAMS
PROTEIN	GRAMS
CALORIES	

SNACK
FAT	GRAMS
CARBS	GRAMS
PROTEIN	GRAMS
CALORIES	

SNACK
FAT	GRAMS
CARBS	GRAMS
PROTEIN	GRAMS
CALORIES	

WATER INTAKE TRACKER

💧 💧 💧 💧 💧 💧 💧 💧

END OF THE DAY TOTAL OVERVIEW

CARBS	FAT	PROTEIN	CALORIES

DAILY TRACKER

DATE _____

SLEEP TRACKER:

☀ RISE: [   ]　　🌙 BEDTIME: [   ]　　💤 SLEEP (HRS): [   ]

EXERCISE			IN A STATE OF KETOSIS?		
TYPE	TIME	DURATION	YES	NO	UNSURE

CRAVINGS			DAILY ENERGY LEVEL		
YES	NO	SOMEWHAT	HIGH	MEDIUM	LOW

MEALS

	BREAKFAST	
	FAT	GRAMS
	CARBS	GRAMS
	PROTEIN	GRAMS
	CALORIES	

	LUNCH	
	FAT	GRAMS
	CARBS	GRAMS
	PROTEIN	GRAMS
	CALORIES	

	DINNER	
	FAT	GRAMS
	CARBS	GRAMS
	PROTEIN	GRAMS
	CALORIES	

	SNACK	
	FAT	GRAMS
	CARBS	GRAMS
	PROTEIN	GRAMS
	CALORIES	

	SNACK	
	FAT	GRAMS
	CARBS	GRAMS
	PROTEIN	GRAMS
	CALORIES	

WATER INTAKE TRACKER

💧 💧 💧 💧 💧 💧 💧 💧

END OF THE DAY TOTAL OVERVIEW

CARBS	FAT	PROTEIN	CALORIES
[ ]	[ ]	[ ]	[ ]

DAILY TRACKER

DATE _____

SLEEP TRACKER:

☀ RISE: [_____]   🌙 zᶻ BEDTIME: [_____]   💭 zᶻ SLEEP (HRS): [_____]

EXERCISE			IN A STATE OF KETOSIS?		
TYPE	TIME	DURATION	YES	NO	UNSURE

CRAVINGS			DAILY ENERGY LEVEL		
YES	NO	SOMEWHAT	HIGH	MEDIUM	LOW

MEALS

	BREAKFAST	
	FAT	GRAMS
	CARBS	GRAMS
	PROTEIN	GRAMS
	CALORIES	

	LUNCH	
	FAT	GRAMS
	CARBS	GRAMS
	PROTEIN	GRAMS
	CALORIES	

	DINNER	
	FAT	GRAMS
	CARBS	GRAMS
	PROTEIN	GRAMS
	CALORIES	

	SNACK	
	FAT	GRAMS
	CARBS	GRAMS
	PROTEIN	GRAMS
	CALORIES	

	SNACK	
	FAT	GRAMS
	CARBS	GRAMS
	PROTEIN	GRAMS
	CALORIES	

WATER INTAKE TRACKER

END OF THE DAY TOTAL OVERVIEW

CARBS	FAT	PROTEIN	CALORIES
[____]	[____]	[____]	[____]

DAILY TRACKER

DATE _____

SLEEP TRACKER:

RISE: [   ] BEDTIME: [   ] SLEEP (HRS): [   ]

EXERCISE			IN A STATE OF KETOSIS?		
TYPE	TIME	DURATION	YES	NO	UNSURE

CRAVINGS			DAILY ENERGY LEVEL		
YES	NO	SOMEWHAT	HIGH	MEDIUM	LOW

MEALS

BREAKFAST

FAT	GRAMS
CARBS	GRAMS
PROTEIN	GRAMS
CALORIES	

LUNCH

FAT	GRAMS
CARBS	GRAMS
PROTEIN	GRAMS
CALORIES	

DINNER

FAT	GRAMS
CARBS	GRAMS
PROTEIN	GRAMS
CALORIES	

SNACK

FAT	GRAMS
CARBS	GRAMS
PROTEIN	GRAMS
CALORIES	

SNACK

FAT	GRAMS
CARBS	GRAMS
PROTEIN	GRAMS
CALORIES	

WATER INTAKE TRACKER

END OF THE DAY TOTAL OVERVIEW

CARBS	FAT	PROTEIN	CALORIES
[ ]	[ ]	[ ]	[ ]

DAILY TRACKER

DATE _____

SLEEP TRACKER:

☼ | RISE: | 🌙 zᶻᶻ | BEDTIME: | 💭zᶻᶻ | SLEEP (HRS):

EXERCISE			IN A STATE OF KETOSIS?		
TYPE	TIME	DURATION	YES	NO	UNSURE

CRAVINGS			DAILY ENERGY LEVEL		
YES	NO	SOMEWHAT	HIGH	MEDIUM	LOW

MEALS

	BREAKFAST	
	FAT	GRAMS
	CARBS	GRAMS
	PROTEIN	GRAMS
	CALORIES	

	LUNCH	
	FAT	GRAMS
	CARBS	GRAMS
	PROTEIN	GRAMS
	CALORIES	

	DINNER	
	FAT	GRAMS
	CARBS	GRAMS
	PROTEIN	GRAMS
	CALORIES	

	SNACK	
	FAT	GRAMS
	CARBS	GRAMS
	PROTEIN	GRAMS
	CALORIES	

	SNACK	
	FAT	GRAMS
	CARBS	GRAMS
	PROTEIN	GRAMS
	CALORIES	

WATER INTAKE TRACKER

💧 💧 💧 💧 💧 💧 💧 💧

END OF THE DAY TOTAL OVERVIEW

CARBS	FAT	PROTEIN	CALORIES

DAILY TRACKER

DATE _____

SLEEP TRACKER:

☀ RISE: _____   🌙 BEDTIME: _____   💤 SLEEP (HRS): _____

EXERCISE			IN A STATE OF KETOSIS?		
TYPE	TIME	DURATION	YES	NO	UNSURE

CRAVINGS			DAILY ENERGY LEVEL		
YES	NO	SOMEWHAT	HIGH	MEDIUM	LOW

MEALS

	BREAKFAST	
	FAT	GRAMS
	CARBS	GRAMS
	PROTEIN	GRAMS
	CALORIES	

	LUNCH	
	FAT	GRAMS
	CARBS	GRAMS
	PROTEIN	GRAMS
	CALORIES	

	DINNER	
	FAT	GRAMS
	CARBS	GRAMS
	PROTEIN	GRAMS
	CALORIES	

	SNACK	
	FAT	GRAMS
	CARBS	GRAMS
	PROTEIN	GRAMS
	CALORIES	

	SNACK	
	FAT	GRAMS
	CARBS	GRAMS
	PROTEIN	GRAMS
	CALORIES	

WATER INTAKE TRACKER

💧 💧 💧 💧 💧 💧 💧 💧

END OF THE DAY TOTAL OVERVIEW

CARBS	FAT	PROTEIN	CALORIES

DAILY TRACKER

DATE _____

SLEEP TRACKER:

☀ | RISE: | 🌙 z z z | BEDTIME: | 💭 z z Z | SLEEP (HRS):

EXERCISE			IN A STATE OF KETOSIS?		
TYPE	TIME	DURATION	YES	NO	UNSURE

CRAVINGS			DAILY ENERGY LEVEL		
YES	NO	SOMEWHAT	HIGH	MEDIUM	LOW

MEALS

	BREAKFAST	
	FAT	GRAMS
	CARBS	GRAMS
	PROTEIN	GRAMS
	CALORIES	

	LUNCH	
	FAT	GRAMS
	CARBS	GRAMS
	PROTEIN	GRAMS
	CALORIES	

	DINNER	
	FAT	GRAMS
	CARBS	GRAMS
	PROTEIN	GRAMS
	CALORIES	

	SNACK	
	FAT	GRAMS
	CARBS	GRAMS
	PROTEIN	GRAMS
	CALORIES	

	SNACK	
	FAT	GRAMS
	CARBS	GRAMS
	PROTEIN	GRAMS
	CALORIES	

WATER INTAKE TRACKER

END OF THE DAY TOTAL OVERVIEW

CARBS	FAT	PROTEIN	CALORIES

DAILY TRACKER

DATE _____

SLEEP TRACKER:

☼ | RISE: | 🌙 | BEDTIME: | 💤 | SLEEP (HRS):

EXERCISE			IN A STATE OF KETOSIS?		
TYPE	TIME	DURATION	YES	NO	UNSURE

CRAVINGS			DAILY ENERGY LEVEL		
YES	NO	SOMEWHAT	HIGH	MEDIUM	LOW

MEALS

BREAKFAST

FAT	GRAMS
CARBS	GRAMS
PROTEIN	GRAMS
CALORIES	

LUNCH

FAT	GRAMS
CARBS	GRAMS
PROTEIN	GRAMS
CALORIES	

DINNER

FAT	GRAMS
CARBS	GRAMS
PROTEIN	GRAMS
CALORIES	

SNACK

FAT	GRAMS
CARBS	GRAMS
PROTEIN	GRAMS
CALORIES	

SNACK

FAT	GRAMS
CARBS	GRAMS
PROTEIN	GRAMS
CALORIES	

WATER INTAKE TRACKER

END OF THE DAY TOTAL OVERVIEW

CARBS	FAT	PROTEIN	CALORIES

DAILY TRACKER

DATE _____

SLEEP TRACKER:

RISE: _____   BEDTIME: _____   SLEEP (HRS): _____

EXERCISE			IN A STATE OF KETOSIS?		
TYPE	TIME	DURATION	YES	NO	UNSURE

CRAVINGS			DAILY ENERGY LEVEL		
YES	NO	SOMEWHAT	HIGH	MEDIUM	LOW

MEALS

	BREAKFAST	
	FAT	GRAMS
	CARBS	GRAMS
	PROTEIN	GRAMS
	CALORIES	

	LUNCH	
	FAT	GRAMS
	CARBS	GRAMS
	PROTEIN	GRAMS
	CALORIES	

	DINNER	
	FAT	GRAMS
	CARBS	GRAMS
	PROTEIN	GRAMS
	CALORIES	

	SNACK	
	FAT	GRAMS
	CARBS	GRAMS
	PROTEIN	GRAMS
	CALORIES	

	SNACK	
	FAT	GRAMS
	CARBS	GRAMS
	PROTEIN	GRAMS
	CALORIES	

WATER INTAKE TRACKER

END OF THE DAY TOTAL OVERVIEW

CARBS	FAT	PROTEIN	CALORIES

DAILY TRACKER

DATE _____

SLEEP TRACKER:

☼ | RISE: | 🌙 zᶻᶻ | BEDTIME: | 💭 | SLEEP (HRS):

EXERCISE			IN A STATE OF KETOSIS?		
TYPE	TIME	DURATION	YES	NO	UNSURE

CRAVINGS			DAILY ENERGY LEVEL		
YES	NO	SOMEWHAT	HIGH	MEDIUM	LOW

MEALS

BREAKFAST
FAT	GRAMS
CARBS	GRAMS
PROTEIN	GRAMS
CALORIES	

LUNCH
FAT	GRAMS
CARBS	GRAMS
PROTEIN	GRAMS
CALORIES	

DINNER
FAT	GRAMS
CARBS	GRAMS
PROTEIN	GRAMS
CALORIES	

SNACK
FAT	GRAMS
CARBS	GRAMS
PROTEIN	GRAMS
CALORIES	

SNACK
FAT	GRAMS
CARBS	GRAMS
PROTEIN	GRAMS
CALORIES	

WATER INTAKE TRACKER

END OF THE DAY TOTAL OVERVIEW

CARBS	FAT	PROTEIN	CALORIES

DAILY TRACKER

DATE _____

SLEEP TRACKER:

☀ RISE: _____   🌙 zᶻᶻ BEDTIME: _____   💭 zᶻᶻ SLEEP (HRS): _____

EXERCISE			IN A STATE OF KETOSIS?		
TYPE	TIME	DURATION	YES	NO	UNSURE

CRAVINGS			DAILY ENERGY LEVEL		
YES	NO	SOMEWHAT	HIGH	MEDIUM	LOW

MEALS

BREAKFAST
FAT	GRAMS
CARBS	GRAMS
PROTEIN	GRAMS
CALORIES	

LUNCH
FAT	GRAMS
CARBS	GRAMS
PROTEIN	GRAMS
CALORIES	

DINNER
FAT	GRAMS
CARBS	GRAMS
PROTEIN	GRAMS
CALORIES	

SNACK
FAT	GRAMS
CARBS	GRAMS
PROTEIN	GRAMS
CALORIES	

SNACK
FAT	GRAMS
CARBS	GRAMS
PROTEIN	GRAMS
CALORIES	

WATER INTAKE TRACKER

END OF THE DAY TOTAL OVERVIEW

CARBS	FAT	PROTEIN	CALORIES

DAILY TRACKER

DATE _____

SLEEP TRACKER:

RISE: _____   BEDTIME: _____   SLEEP (HRS): _____

EXERCISE			IN A STATE OF KETOSIS?		
TYPE	TIME	DURATION	YES	NO	UNSURE

CRAVINGS			DAILY ENERGY LEVEL		
YES	NO	SOMEWHAT	HIGH	MEDIUM	LOW

MEALS

BREAKFAST

FAT	GRAMS
CARBS	GRAMS
PROTEIN	GRAMS
CALORIES	

LUNCH

FAT	GRAMS
CARBS	GRAMS
PROTEIN	GRAMS
CALORIES	

DINNER

FAT	GRAMS
CARBS	GRAMS
PROTEIN	GRAMS
CALORIES	

SNACK

FAT	GRAMS
CARBS	GRAMS
PROTEIN	GRAMS
CALORIES	

SNACK

FAT	GRAMS
CARBS	GRAMS
PROTEIN	GRAMS
CALORIES	

WATER INTAKE TRACKER

END OF THE DAY TOTAL OVERVIEW

CARBS	FAT	PROTEIN	CALORIES

DAILY TRACKER

DATE _____

SLEEP TRACKER:

RISE: _____   BEDTIME: _____   SLEEP (HRS): _____

EXERCISE			IN A STATE OF KETOSIS?		
TYPE	TIME	DURATION	YES	NO	UNSURE

CRAVINGS			DAILY ENERGY LEVEL		
YES	NO	SOMEWHAT	HIGH	MEDIUM	LOW

MEALS

BREAKFAST
FAT	GRAMS
CARBS	GRAMS
PROTEIN	GRAMS
CALORIES	

LUNCH
FAT	GRAMS
CARBS	GRAMS
PROTEIN	GRAMS
CALORIES	

DINNER
FAT	GRAMS
CARBS	GRAMS
PROTEIN	GRAMS
CALORIES	

SNACK
FAT	GRAMS
CARBS	GRAMS
PROTEIN	GRAMS
CALORIES	

SNACK
FAT	GRAMS
CARBS	GRAMS
PROTEIN	GRAMS
CALORIES	

WATER INTAKE TRACKER

END OF THE DAY TOTAL OVERVIEW

CARBS	FAT	PROTEIN	CALORIES

DAILY TRACKER

DATE _____

SLEEP TRACKER:

☀ RISE: _____   🌙 BEDTIME: _____   💤 SLEEP (HRS): _____

EXERCISE
TYPE   TIME   DURATION

IN A STATE OF KETOSIS?
YES   NO   UNSURE

CRAVINGS
YES   NO   SOMEWHAT

DAILY ENERGY LEVEL
HIGH   MEDIUM   LOW

MEALS

	BREAKFAST	
	FAT	GRAMS
	CARBS	GRAMS
	PROTEIN	GRAMS
	CALORIES	

	LUNCH	
	FAT	GRAMS
	CARBS	GRAMS
	PROTEIN	GRAMS
	CALORIES	

	DINNER	
	FAT	GRAMS
	CARBS	GRAMS
	PROTEIN	GRAMS
	CALORIES	

	SNACK	
	FAT	GRAMS
	CARBS	GRAMS
	PROTEIN	GRAMS
	CALORIES	

	SNACK	
	FAT	GRAMS
	CARBS	GRAMS
	PROTEIN	GRAMS
	CALORIES	

WATER INTAKE TRACKER

END OF THE DAY TOTAL OVERVIEW

CARBS	FAT	PROTEIN	CALORIES

DAILY TRACKER

DATE _____

SLEEP TRACKER:

☀ | RISE: | 🌙 | BEDTIME: | 💭 | SLEEP (HRS):

EXERCISE			IN A STATE OF KETOSIS?		
TYPE	TIME	DURATION	YES	NO	UNSURE

CRAVINGS			DAILY ENERGY LEVEL		
YES	NO	SOMEWHAT	HIGH	MEDIUM	LOW

MEALS

	BREAKFAST	
	FAT	GRAMS
	CARBS	GRAMS
	PROTEIN	GRAMS
	CALORIES	

	LUNCH	
	FAT	GRAMS
	CARBS	GRAMS
	PROTEIN	GRAMS
	CALORIES	

	DINNER	
	FAT	GRAMS
	CARBS	GRAMS
	PROTEIN	GRAMS
	CALORIES	

	SNACK	
	FAT	GRAMS
	CARBS	GRAMS
	PROTEIN	GRAMS
	CALORIES	

	SNACK	
	FAT	GRAMS
	CARBS	GRAMS
	PROTEIN	GRAMS
	CALORIES	

WATER INTAKE TRACKER

END OF THE DAY TOTAL OVERVIEW

CARBS	FAT	PROTEIN	CALORIES

DAILY TRACKER

DATE _____

SLEEP TRACKER:

☀ RISE: _____   🌙 zzz BEDTIME: _____   💤 SLEEP (HRS): _____

EXERCISE			IN A STATE OF KETOSIS?		
TYPE	TIME	DURATION	YES	NO	UNSURE

CRAVINGS			DAILY ENERGY LEVEL		
YES	NO	SOMEWHAT	HIGH	MEDIUM	LOW

MEALS

BREAKFAST

FAT	GRAMS
CARBS	GRAMS
PROTEIN	GRAMS
CALORIES	

LUNCH

FAT	GRAMS
CARBS	GRAMS
PROTEIN	GRAMS
CALORIES	

DINNER

FAT	GRAMS
CARBS	GRAMS
PROTEIN	GRAMS
CALORIES	

SNACK

FAT	GRAMS
CARBS	GRAMS
PROTEIN	GRAMS
CALORIES	

SNACK

FAT	GRAMS
CARBS	GRAMS
PROTEIN	GRAMS
CALORIES	

WATER INTAKE TRACKER

💧 💧 💧 💧 💧 💧 💧 💧

END OF THE DAY TOTAL OVERVIEW

CARBS	FAT	PROTEIN	CALORIES

DAILY TRACKER

DATE _____

SLEEP TRACKER:

☀ | RISE: | 🌙 z z z | BEDTIME: | 💤 | SLEEP (HRS):

EXERCISE			IN A STATE OF KETOSIS?		
TYPE	TIME	DURATION	YES	NO	UNSURE

CRAVINGS			DAILY ENERGY LEVEL		
YES	NO	SOMEWHAT	HIGH	MEDIUM	LOW

MEALS

BREAKFAST
FAT		GRAMS
CARBS		GRAMS
PROTEIN		GRAMS
CALORIES		

LUNCH
FAT		GRAMS
CARBS		GRAMS
PROTEIN		GRAMS
CALORIES		

DINNER
FAT		GRAMS
CARBS		GRAMS
PROTEIN		GRAMS
CALORIES		

SNACK
FAT		GRAMS
CARBS		GRAMS
PROTEIN		GRAMS
CALORIES		

SNACK
FAT		GRAMS
CARBS		GRAMS
PROTEIN		GRAMS
CALORIES		

WATER INTAKE TRACKER

END OF THE DAY TOTAL OVERVIEW

CARBS	FAT	PROTEIN	CALORIES

DAILY TRACKER

DATE _____

SLEEP TRACKER:

☼ | RISE: | 🌙 | BEDTIME: | 💤 | SLEEP (HRS):

EXERCISE			IN A STATE OF KETOSIS?		
TYPE	TIME	DURATION	YES	NO	UNSURE

CRAVINGS			DAILY ENERGY LEVEL		
YES	NO	SOMEWHAT	HIGH	MEDIUM	LOW

MEALS

	BREAKFAST	
	FAT	GRAMS
	CARBS	GRAMS
	PROTEIN	GRAMS
	CALORIES	

	LUNCH	
	FAT	GRAMS
	CARBS	GRAMS
	PROTEIN	GRAMS
	CALORIES	

	DINNER	
	FAT	GRAMS
	CARBS	GRAMS
	PROTEIN	GRAMS
	CALORIES	

	SNACK	
	FAT	GRAMS
	CARBS	GRAMS
	PROTEIN	GRAMS
	CALORIES	

	SNACK	
	FAT	GRAMS
	CARBS	GRAMS
	PROTEIN	GRAMS
	CALORIES	

WATER INTAKE TRACKER

END OF THE DAY TOTAL OVERVIEW

CARBS	FAT	PROTEIN	CALORIES

DAILY TRACKER

DATE _____

SLEEP TRACKER:

☀ RISE: _____   🌙 zzz BEDTIME: _____   💤 SLEEP (HRS): _____

EXERCISE			IN A STATE OF KETOSIS?		
TYPE	TIME	DURATION	YES	NO	UNSURE

CRAVINGS			DAILY ENERGY LEVEL		
YES	NO	SOMEWHAT	HIGH	MEDIUM	LOW

MEALS

BREAKFAST
FAT	GRAMS
CARBS	GRAMS
PROTEIN	GRAMS
CALORIES	

LUNCH
FAT	GRAMS
CARBS	GRAMS
PROTEIN	GRAMS
CALORIES	

DINNER
FAT	GRAMS
CARBS	GRAMS
PROTEIN	GRAMS
CALORIES	

SNACK
FAT	GRAMS
CARBS	GRAMS
PROTEIN	GRAMS
CALORIES	

SNACK
FAT	GRAMS
CARBS	GRAMS
PROTEIN	GRAMS
CALORIES	

WATER INTAKE TRACKER

END OF THE DAY TOTAL OVERVIEW

CARBS	FAT	PROTEIN	CALORIES

DAILY TRACKER

DATE _____

SLEEP TRACKER:

☀ | RISE: _____ | 🌙 zzz | BEDTIME: _____ | 💭zzz | SLEEP (HRS): _____

EXERCISE			IN A STATE OF KETOSIS?		
TYPE	TIME	DURATION	YES	NO	UNSURE

CRAVINGS			DAILY ENERGY LEVEL		
YES	NO	SOMEWHAT	HIGH	MEDIUM	LOW

MEALS

	BREAKFAST	
	FAT	GRAMS
	CARBS	GRAMS
	PROTEIN	GRAMS
	CALORIES	

	LUNCH	
	FAT	GRAMS
	CARBS	GRAMS
	PROTEIN	GRAMS
	CALORIES	

	DINNER	
	FAT	GRAMS
	CARBS	GRAMS
	PROTEIN	GRAMS
	CALORIES	

	SNACK	
	FAT	GRAMS
	CARBS	GRAMS
	PROTEIN	GRAMS
	CALORIES	

	SNACK	
	FAT	GRAMS
	CARBS	GRAMS
	PROTEIN	GRAMS
	CALORIES	

WATER INTAKE TRACKER

💧 💧 💧 💧 💧 💧 💧 💧

END OF THE DAY TOTAL OVERVIEW

CARBS	FAT	PROTEIN	CALORIES

DAILY TRACKER

DATE _____

SLEEP TRACKER:

| RISE: | | BEDTIME: | | SLEEP (HRS): |

EXERCISE

TYPE   TIME   DURATION

IN A STATE OF KETOSIS?

YES   NO   UNSURE

CRAVINGS

YES   NO   SOMEWHAT

DAILY ENERGY LEVEL

HIGH   MEDIUM   LOW

MEALS

BREAKFAST
FAT		GRAMS
CARBS		GRAMS
PROTEIN		GRAMS
CALORIES		

LUNCH
FAT		GRAMS
CARBS		GRAMS
PROTEIN		GRAMS
CALORIES		

DINNER
FAT		GRAMS
CARBS		GRAMS
PROTEIN		GRAMS
CALORIES		

SNACK
FAT		GRAMS
CARBS		GRAMS
PROTEIN		GRAMS
CALORIES		

SNACK
FAT		GRAMS
CARBS		GRAMS
PROTEIN		GRAMS
CALORIES		

WATER INTAKE TRACKER

END OF THE DAY TOTAL OVERVIEW

CARBS	FAT	PROTEIN	CALORIES

DAILY TRACKER

DATE _____

SLEEP TRACKER:

☀ | RISE: | 🌙 | BEDTIME: | 💭 | SLEEP (HRS):

EXERCISE			IN A STATE OF KETOSIS?		
TYPE	TIME	DURATION	YES	NO	UNSURE

CRAVINGS			DAILY ENERGY LEVEL		
YES	NO	SOMEWHAT	HIGH	MEDIUM	LOW

MEALS

BREAKFAST
FAT   GRAMS
CARBS   GRAMS
PROTEIN   GRAMS
CALORIES

LUNCH
FAT   GRAMS
CARBS   GRAMS
PROTEIN   GRAMS
CALORIES

DINNER
FAT   GRAMS
CARBS   GRAMS
PROTEIN   GRAMS
CALORIES

SNACK
FAT   GRAMS
CARBS   GRAMS
PROTEIN   GRAMS
CALORIES

SNACK
FAT   GRAMS
CARBS   GRAMS
PROTEIN   GRAMS
CALORIES

WATER INTAKE TRACKER

💧 💧 💧 💧 💧 💧 💧 💧

END OF THE DAY TOTAL OVERVIEW

CARBS	FAT	PROTEIN	CALORIES

INTERMITTENT FASTING

DATES:

	START TIME	END TIME	TOTAL HOURS
MON			
TUE	:	:	
WED	:	:	
THU	;	;	
FRI	:	:	
SAT	:	:	
SUN	:	:	

DATES:

	START TIME	END TIME	TOTAL HOURS
MON			
TUE	:	:	
WED	:	:	
THU	;	;	
FRI	:	:	
SAT	:	:	
SUN	:	:	

DATES:

	START TIME	END TIME	TOTAL HOURS
MON			
TUE	:	:	
WED	:	:	
THU	;	;	
FRI	:	:	
SAT	:	:	
SUN	:	:	

DATES:

	START TIME	END TIME	TOTAL HOURS
MON			
TUE	:	:	
WED	:	:	
THU	;	;	
FRI	:	:	
SAT	:	:	
SUN	:	:	

DATES:

	START TIME	END TIME	TOTAL HOURS
MON			
TUE	:	:	
WED	:	:	
THU	;	;	
FRI	:	:	
SAT	:	:	
SUN	:	:	

DATES:

	START TIME	END TIME	TOTAL HOURS
MON			
TUE	:	:	
WED	:	:	
THU	;	;	
FRI	:	:	
SAT	:	:	
SUN	:	:	

DATES:

	START TIME	END TIME	TOTAL HOURS
MON			
TUE	:	:	
WED	:	:	
THU	;	;	
FRI	:	:	
SAT	:	:	
SUN	:	:	

DATES:

	START TIME	END TIME	TOTAL HOURS
MON			
TUE	:	:	
WED	:	:	
THU	;	;	
FRI	:	:	
SAT	:	:	
SUN	:	:	

DATES:

	START TIME	END TIME	TOTAL HOURS
MON			
TUE	:	:	
WED	:	:	
THU	;	;	
FRI	:	:	
SAT	:	:	
SUN	:	:	

NOTES

INTERMITTENT FASTING

DATES:	START TIME	END TIME	TOTAL HOURS
MON			
TUE	:	:	
WED	:	:	
THU	;	;	
FRI	:	:	
SAT	:	:	
SUN	:	:	

DATES:	START TIME	END TIME	TOTAL HOURS
MON			
TUE	:	:	
WED	:	:	
THU	;	;	
FRI	:	:	
SAT	:	:	
SUN	:	:	

DATES:	START TIME	END TIME	TOTAL HOURS
MON			
TUE	:	:	
WED	:	:	
THU	;	;	
FRI	:	:	
SAT	:	:	
SUN	:	:	

DATES:	START TIME	END TIME	TOTAL HOURS
MON			
TUE	:	:	
WED	:	:	
THU	;	;	
FRI	:	:	
SAT	:	:	
SUN	:	:	

DATES:	START TIME	END TIME	TOTAL HOURS
MON			
TUE	:	:	
WED	:	:	
THU	;	;	
FRI	:	:	
SAT	:	:	
SUN	:	:	

DATES:	START TIME	END TIME	TOTAL HOURS
MON			
TUE	:	:	
WED	:	:	
THU	;	;	
FRI	:	:	
SAT	:	:	
SUN	:	:	

DATES:	START TIME	END TIME	TOTAL HOURS
MON			
TUE	:	:	
WED	:	:	
THU	;	;	
FRI	:	:	
SAT	:	:	
SUN	:	:	

DATES:	START TIME	END TIME	TOTAL HOURS
MON			
TUE	:	:	
WED	:	:	
THU	;	;	
FRI	:	:	
SAT	:	:	
SUN	:	:	

DATES:	START TIME	END TIME	TOTAL HOURS
MON			
TUE	:	:	
WED	:	:	
THU	;	;	
FRI	:	:	
SAT	:	:	
SUN	:	:	

NOTES

60 DAYS OF KETO

STARTING WEIGHT: **DAY 60 WEIGHT:**

1	2	3	4	5	6	7	8	9	10	LBS LOST: INCHES LOST:
11	12	13	14	15	16	17	18	19	20	LBS LOST: INCHES LOST:
21	22	23	24	25	26	27	28	29	30	LBS LOST: INCHES LOST:
31	32	33	34	35	36	37	38	39	40	LBS LOST: INCHES LOST:
41	42	43	44	45	46	47	48	49	50	LBS LOST: INCHES LOST:
51	52	53	54	55	56	57	58	59	60	LBS LOST: INCHES LOST:

TOTAL WEIGHT LOST: **TOTAL INCHES LOST:**

THOUGHTS & REFLECTIONS:

DAILY TRACKER

DATE _____

SLEEP TRACKER:

RISE: _____   BEDTIME: _____   SLEEP (HRS): _____

EXERCISE			IN A STATE OF KETOSIS?		
TYPE	TIME	DURATION	YES	NO	UNSURE

CRAVINGS			DAILY ENERGY LEVEL		
YES	NO	SOMEWHAT	HIGH	MEDIUM	LOW

MEALS

BREAKFAST
FAT	GRAMS
CARBS	GRAMS
PROTEIN	GRAMS
CALORIES	

LUNCH
FAT	GRAMS
CARBS	GRAMS
PROTEIN	GRAMS
CALORIES	

DINNER
FAT	GRAMS
CARBS	GRAMS
PROTEIN	GRAMS
CALORIES	

SNACK
FAT	GRAMS
CARBS	GRAMS
PROTEIN	GRAMS
CALORIES	

SNACK
FAT	GRAMS
CARBS	GRAMS
PROTEIN	GRAMS
CALORIES	

WATER INTAKE TRACKER

END OF THE DAY TOTAL OVERVIEW

CARBS	FAT	PROTEIN	CALORIES

DAILY TRACKER

DATE _____

SLEEP TRACKER:

☀ RISE: _____ 🌙 zzz BEDTIME: _____ 💭zZZ SLEEP (HRS): _____

EXERCISE

TYPE	TIME	DURATION

IN A STATE OF KETOSIS?

YES   NO   UNSURE

CRAVINGS

YES   NO   SOMEWHAT

DAILY ENERGY LEVEL

HIGH   MEDIUM   LOW

MEALS

BREAKFAST
FAT		GRAMS
CARBS		GRAMS
PROTEIN		GRAMS
CALORIES		

LUNCH
FAT		GRAMS
CARBS		GRAMS
PROTEIN		GRAMS
CALORIES		

DINNER
FAT		GRAMS
CARBS		GRAMS
PROTEIN		GRAMS
CALORIES		

SNACK
FAT		GRAMS
CARBS		GRAMS
PROTEIN		GRAMS
CALORIES		

SNACK
FAT		GRAMS
CARBS		GRAMS
PROTEIN		GRAMS
CALORIES		

WATER INTAKE TRACKER

💧 💧 💧 💧 💧 💧 💧 💧

END OF THE DAY TOTAL OVERVIEW

CARBS	FAT	PROTEIN	CALORIES

DAILY TRACKER

DATE _____

SLEEP TRACKER:

☀ RISE: _____   🌙 BEDTIME: _____   💤 SLEEP (HRS): _____

EXERCISE			IN A STATE OF KETOSIS?		
TYPE	TIME	DURATION	YES	NO	UNSURE

CRAVINGS			DAILY ENERGY LEVEL		
YES	NO	SOMEWHAT	HIGH	MEDIUM	LOW

MEALS

BREAKFAST
FAT	GRAMS
CARBS	GRAMS
PROTEIN	GRAMS
CALORIES	

LUNCH
FAT	GRAMS
CARBS	GRAMS
PROTEIN	GRAMS
CALORIES	

DINNER
FAT	GRAMS
CARBS	GRAMS
PROTEIN	GRAMS
CALORIES	

SNACK
FAT	GRAMS
CARBS	GRAMS
PROTEIN	GRAMS
CALORIES	

SNACK
FAT	GRAMS
CARBS	GRAMS
PROTEIN	GRAMS
CALORIES	

WATER INTAKE TRACKER

END OF THE DAY TOTAL OVERVIEW

CARBS	FAT	PROTEIN	CALORIES

DAILY TRACKER

DATE _____

SLEEP TRACKER:

☀ RISE: _____   🌙 zzz BEDTIME: _____   💭zzZ SLEEP (HRS): _____

EXERCISE			IN A STATE OF KETOSIS?		
TYPE	TIME	DURATION	YES	NO	UNSURE

CRAVINGS			DAILY ENERGY LEVEL		
YES	NO	SOMEWHAT	HIGH	MEDIUM	LOW

MEALS

	BREAKFAST	
	FAT	GRAMS
	CARBS	GRAMS
	PROTEIN	GRAMS
	CALORIES	

	LUNCH	
	FAT	GRAMS
	CARBS	GRAMS
	PROTEIN	GRAMS
	CALORIES	

	DINNER	
	FAT	GRAMS
	CARBS	GRAMS
	PROTEIN	GRAMS
	CALORIES	

	SNACK	
	FAT	GRAMS
	CARBS	GRAMS
	PROTEIN	GRAMS
	CALORIES	

	SNACK	
	FAT	GRAMS
	CARBS	GRAMS
	PROTEIN	GRAMS
	CALORIES	

WATER INTAKE TRACKER

💧 💧 💧 💧 💧 💧 💧 💧

END OF THE DAY TOTAL OVERVIEW

CARBS	FAT	PROTEIN	CALORIES
_____	_____	_____	_____

DAILY TRACKER

DATE _____

SLEEP TRACKER:

☀ | RISE: | 🌙 | BEDTIME: | 💭 | SLEEP (HRS):

EXERCISE			IN A STATE OF KETOSIS?		
TYPE	TIME	DURATION	YES	NO	UNSURE

CRAVINGS			DAILY ENERGY LEVEL		
YES	NO	SOMEWHAT	HIGH	MEDIUM	LOW

MEALS

BREAKFAST
FAT		GRAMS
CARBS		GRAMS
PROTEIN		GRAMS
CALORIES		

LUNCH
FAT		GRAMS
CARBS		GRAMS
PROTEIN		GRAMS
CALORIES		

DINNER
FAT		GRAMS
CARBS		GRAMS
PROTEIN		GRAMS
CALORIES		

SNACK
FAT		GRAMS
CARBS		GRAMS
PROTEIN		GRAMS
CALORIES		

SNACK
FAT		GRAMS
CARBS		GRAMS
PROTEIN		GRAMS
CALORIES		

WATER INTAKE TRACKER

END OF THE DAY TOTAL OVERVIEW

CARBS	FAT	PROTEIN	CALORIES

DAILY TRACKER

DATE _____

SLEEP TRACKER:

RISE: _____   BEDTIME: _____   SLEEP (HRS): _____

EXERCISE			IN A STATE OF KETOSIS?		
TYPE	TIME	DURATION	YES	NO	UNSURE

CRAVINGS			DAILY ENERGY LEVEL		
YES	NO	SOMEWHAT	HIGH	MEDIUM	LOW

MEALS

BREAKFAST
FAT		GRAMS
CARBS		GRAMS
PROTEIN		GRAMS
CALORIES		

LUNCH
FAT		GRAMS
CARBS		GRAMS
PROTEIN		GRAMS
CALORIES		

DINNER
FAT		GRAMS
CARBS		GRAMS
PROTEIN		GRAMS
CALORIES		

SNACK
FAT		GRAMS
CARBS		GRAMS
PROTEIN		GRAMS
CALORIES		

SNACK
FAT		GRAMS
CARBS		GRAMS
PROTEIN		GRAMS
CALORIES		

WATER INTAKE TRACKER

END OF THE DAY TOTAL OVERVIEW

CARBS	FAT	PROTEIN	CALORIES

DAILY TRACKER

DATE _____

SLEEP TRACKER:

☀ RISE: _____ 🌙 BEDTIME: _____ 💤 SLEEP (HRS): _____

EXERCISE			IN A STATE OF KETOSIS?		
TYPE	TIME	DURATION	YES	NO	UNSURE

CRAVINGS			DAILY ENERGY LEVEL		
YES	NO	SOMEWHAT	HIGH	MEDIUM	LOW

MEALS

BREAKFAST
FAT	GRAMS
CARBS	GRAMS
PROTEIN	GRAMS
CALORIES	

LUNCH
FAT	GRAMS
CARBS	GRAMS
PROTEIN	GRAMS
CALORIES	

DINNER
FAT	GRAMS
CARBS	GRAMS
PROTEIN	GRAMS
CALORIES	

SNACK
FAT	GRAMS
CARBS	GRAMS
PROTEIN	GRAMS
CALORIES	

SNACK
FAT	GRAMS
CARBS	GRAMS
PROTEIN	GRAMS
CALORIES	

WATER INTAKE TRACKER

END OF THE DAY TOTAL OVERVIEW

CARBS	FAT	PROTEIN	CALORIES

DAILY TRACKER

DATE _____

SLEEP TRACKER:

☀ RISE: _____   🌙 z z z BEDTIME: _____   💤 z z z SLEEP (HRS): _____

EXERCISE			IN A STATE OF KETOSIS?		
TYPE	TIME	DURATION	YES	NO	UNSURE

CRAVINGS			DAILY ENERGY LEVEL		
YES	NO	SOMEWHAT	HIGH	MEDIUM	LOW

MEALS

	BREAKFAST	
	FAT	GRAMS
	CARBS	GRAMS
	PROTEIN	GRAMS
	CALORIES	

	LUNCH	
	FAT	GRAMS
	CARBS	GRAMS
	PROTEIN	GRAMS
	CALORIES	

	DINNER	
	FAT	GRAMS
	CARBS	GRAMS
	PROTEIN	GRAMS
	CALORIES	

	SNACK	
	FAT	GRAMS
	CARBS	GRAMS
	PROTEIN	GRAMS
	CALORIES	

	SNACK	
	FAT	GRAMS
	CARBS	GRAMS
	PROTEIN	GRAMS
	CALORIES	

WATER INTAKE TRACKER

END OF THE DAY TOTAL OVERVIEW

CARBS	FAT	PROTEIN	CALORIES

DAILY TRACKER

DATE _____

SLEEP TRACKER:

☀ | RISE: | 🌙 | BEDTIME: | 💤 | SLEEP (HRS):

EXERCISE			IN A STATE OF KETOSIS?		
TYPE	TIME	DURATION	YES	NO	UNSURE

CRAVINGS			DAILY ENERGY LEVEL		
YES	NO	SOMEWHAT	HIGH	MEDIUM	LOW

MEALS

	BREAKFAST	
	FAT	GRAMS
	CARBS	GRAMS
	PROTEIN	GRAMS
	CALORIES	

	LUNCH	
	FAT	GRAMS
	CARBS	GRAMS
	PROTEIN	GRAMS
	CALORIES	

	DINNER	
	FAT	GRAMS
	CARBS	GRAMS
	PROTEIN	GRAMS
	CALORIES	

	SNACK	
	FAT	GRAMS
	CARBS	GRAMS
	PROTEIN	GRAMS
	CALORIES	

	SNACK	
	FAT	GRAMS
	CARBS	GRAMS
	PROTEIN	GRAMS
	CALORIES	

WATER INTAKE TRACKER

💧 💧 💧 💧 💧 💧 💧 💧

END OF THE DAY TOTAL OVERVIEW

CARBS	FAT	PROTEIN	CALORIES

DAILY TRACKER

DATE _____

SLEEP TRACKER:

RISE: _____   BEDTIME: _____   SLEEP (HRS): _____

EXERCISE			IN A STATE OF KETOSIS?		
TYPE	TIME	DURATION	YES	NO	UNSURE

CRAVINGS			DAILY ENERGY LEVEL		
YES	NO	SOMEWHAT	HIGH	MEDIUM	LOW

MEALS

BREAKFAST
FAT	GRAMS
CARBS	GRAMS
PROTEIN	GRAMS
CALORIES	

LUNCH
FAT	GRAMS
CARBS	GRAMS
PROTEIN	GRAMS
CALORIES	

DINNER
FAT	GRAMS
CARBS	GRAMS
PROTEIN	GRAMS
CALORIES	

SNACK
FAT	GRAMS
CARBS	GRAMS
PROTEIN	GRAMS
CALORIES	

SNACK
FAT	GRAMS
CARBS	GRAMS
PROTEIN	GRAMS
CALORIES	

WATER INTAKE TRACKER

END OF THE DAY TOTAL OVERVIEW

CARBS	FAT	PROTEIN	CALORIES

DAILY TRACKER

DATE _____

SLEEP TRACKER:

RISE: | BEDTIME: | SLEEP (HRS):

EXERCISE
TYPE   TIME   DURATION

IN A STATE OF KETOSIS?
YES   NO   UNSURE

CRAVINGS
YES   NO   SOMEWHAT

DAILY ENERGY LEVEL
HIGH   MEDIUM   LOW

MEALS

	BREAKFAST	
FAT		GRAMS
CARBS		GRAMS
PROTEIN		GRAMS
CALORIES		

	LUNCH	
FAT		GRAMS
CARBS		GRAMS
PROTEIN		GRAMS
CALORIES		

	DINNER	
FAT		GRAMS
CARBS		GRAMS
PROTEIN		GRAMS
CALORIES		

	SNACK	
FAT		GRAMS
CARBS		GRAMS
PROTEIN		GRAMS
CALORIES		

	SNACK	
FAT		GRAMS
CARBS		GRAMS
PROTEIN		GRAMS
CALORIES		

WATER INTAKE TRACKER

END OF THE DAY TOTAL OVERVIEW

CARBS	FAT	PROTEIN	CALORIES

DAILY TRACKER

DATE _____

SLEEP TRACKER:

☼ | RISE: | 🌙 z_z^z | BEDTIME: | 💭 | SLEEP (HRS):

EXERCISE			IN A STATE OF KETOSIS?		
TYPE	TIME	DURATION	YES	NO	UNSURE

CRAVINGS			DAILY ENERGY LEVEL		
YES	NO	SOMEWHAT	HIGH	MEDIUM	LOW

MEALS

	BREAKFAST	
	FAT	GRAMS
	CARBS	GRAMS
	PROTEIN	GRAMS
	CALORIES	

	LUNCH	
	FAT	GRAMS
	CARBS	GRAMS
	PROTEIN	GRAMS
	CALORIES	

	DINNER	
	FAT	GRAMS
	CARBS	GRAMS
	PROTEIN	GRAMS
	CALORIES	

	SNACK	
	FAT	GRAMS
	CARBS	GRAMS
	PROTEIN	GRAMS
	CALORIES	

	SNACK	
	FAT	GRAMS
	CARBS	GRAMS
	PROTEIN	GRAMS
	CALORIES	

WATER INTAKE TRACKER

💧 💧 💧 💧 💧 💧 💧 💧

END OF THE DAY TOTAL OVERVIEW

CARBS	FAT	PROTEIN	CALORIES

DAILY TRACKER

DATE _____

SLEEP TRACKER:

☼ RISE: [   ]   🌙 BEDTIME: [   ]   💭 SLEEP (HRS): [   ]

EXERCISE			IN A STATE OF KETOSIS?		
TYPE	TIME	DURATION	YES	NO	UNSURE

CRAVINGS			DAILY ENERGY LEVEL		
YES	NO	SOMEWHAT	HIGH	MEDIUM	LOW

MEALS

	BREAKFAST	
	FAT	GRAMS
	CARBS	GRAMS
	PROTEIN	GRAMS
	CALORIES	

	LUNCH	
	FAT	GRAMS
	CARBS	GRAMS
	PROTEIN	GRAMS
	CALORIES	

	DINNER	
	FAT	GRAMS
	CARBS	GRAMS
	PROTEIN	GRAMS
	CALORIES	

	SNACK	
	FAT	GRAMS
	CARBS	GRAMS
	PROTEIN	GRAMS
	CALORIES	

	SNACK	
	FAT	GRAMS
	CARBS	GRAMS
	PROTEIN	GRAMS
	CALORIES	

WATER INTAKE TRACKER

💧 💧 💧 💧 💧 💧 💧 💧

END OF THE DAY TOTAL OVERVIEW

CARBS	FAT	PROTEIN	CALORIES
[ ]	[ ]	[ ]	[ ]

DAILY TRACKER

DATE _____

SLEEP TRACKER:

☀ RISE: _____ 🌙 ᶻᶻᶻ BEDTIME: _____ 💭 ᶻᶻᶻ SLEEP (HRS): _____

EXERCISE			IN A STATE OF KETOSIS?		
TYPE	TIME	DURATION	YES	NO	UNSURE

CRAVINGS			DAILY ENERGY LEVEL		
YES	NO	SOMEWHAT	HIGH	MEDIUM	LOW

MEALS

BREAKFAST
FAT	GRAMS
CARBS	GRAMS
PROTEIN	GRAMS
CALORIES	

LUNCH
FAT	GRAMS
CARBS	GRAMS
PROTEIN	GRAMS
CALORIES	

DINNER
FAT	GRAMS
CARBS	GRAMS
PROTEIN	GRAMS
CALORIES	

SNACK
FAT	GRAMS
CARBS	GRAMS
PROTEIN	GRAMS
CALORIES	

SNACK
FAT	GRAMS
CARBS	GRAMS
PROTEIN	GRAMS
CALORIES	

WATER INTAKE TRACKER

END OF THE DAY TOTAL OVERVIEW

CARBS	FAT	PROTEIN	CALORIES

DAILY TRACKER

DATE _____

SLEEP TRACKER:

RISE: _____ BEDTIME: _____ SLEEP (HRS): _____

EXERCISE
TYPE   TIME   DURATION

IN A STATE OF KETOSIS?
YES   NO   UNSURE

CRAVINGS
YES   NO   SOMEWHAT

DAILY ENERGY LEVEL
HIGH   MEDIUM   LOW

MEALS

	BREAKFAST	
	FAT	GRAMS
	CARBS	GRAMS
	PROTEIN	GRAMS
	CALORIES	

	LUNCH	
	FAT	GRAMS
	CARBS	GRAMS
	PROTEIN	GRAMS
	CALORIES	

	DINNER	
	FAT	GRAMS
	CARBS	GRAMS
	PROTEIN	GRAMS
	CALORIES	

	SNACK	
	FAT	GRAMS
	CARBS	GRAMS
	PROTEIN	GRAMS
	CALORIES	

	SNACK	
	FAT	GRAMS
	CARBS	GRAMS
	PROTEIN	GRAMS
	CALORIES	

WATER INTAKE TRACKER

END OF THE DAY TOTAL OVERVIEW

CARBS   FAT   PROTEIN   CALORIES

DAILY TRACKER

DATE _____

SLEEP TRACKER:

☀ | RISE: | 🌙 | BEDTIME: | 💤 | SLEEP (HRS):

EXERCISE			IN A STATE OF KETOSIS?		
TYPE	TIME	DURATION	YES	NO	UNSURE

CRAVINGS			DAILY ENERGY LEVEL		
YES	NO	SOMEWHAT	HIGH	MEDIUM	LOW

MEALS

BREAKFAST
FAT	GRAMS
CARBS	GRAMS
PROTEIN	GRAMS
CALORIES	

LUNCH
FAT	GRAMS
CARBS	GRAMS
PROTEIN	GRAMS
CALORIES	

DINNER
FAT	GRAMS
CARBS	GRAMS
PROTEIN	GRAMS
CALORIES	

SNACK
FAT	GRAMS
CARBS	GRAMS
PROTEIN	GRAMS
CALORIES	

SNACK
FAT	GRAMS
CARBS	GRAMS
PROTEIN	GRAMS
CALORIES	

WATER INTAKE TRACKER

END OF THE DAY TOTAL OVERVIEW

CARBS	FAT	PROTEIN	CALORIES

DAILY TRACKER

DATE _____

SLEEP TRACKER:

RISE: [   ]   BEDTIME: [   ]   SLEEP (HRS): [   ]

EXERCISE			IN A STATE OF KETOSIS?		
TYPE	TIME	DURATION	YES	NO	UNSURE

CRAVINGS			DAILY ENERGY LEVEL		
YES	NO	SOMEWHAT	HIGH	MEDIUM	LOW

MEALS

	BREAKFAST	
	FAT	GRAMS
	CARBS	GRAMS
	PROTEIN	GRAMS
	CALORIES	

	LUNCH	
	FAT	GRAMS
	CARBS	GRAMS
	PROTEIN	GRAMS
	CALORIES	

	DINNER	
	FAT	GRAMS
	CARBS	GRAMS
	PROTEIN	GRAMS
	CALORIES	

	SNACK	
	FAT	GRAMS
	CARBS	GRAMS
	PROTEIN	GRAMS
	CALORIES	

	SNACK	
	FAT	GRAMS
	CARBS	GRAMS
	PROTEIN	GRAMS
	CALORIES	

WATER INTAKE TRACKER

END OF THE DAY TOTAL OVERVIEW

CARBS	FAT	PROTEIN	CALORIES
[ ]	[ ]	[ ]	[ ]

DAILY TRACKER

DATE _____

SLEEP TRACKER:

☀ | RISE: | 🌙 ᶻᶻᶻ | BEDTIME: | 💭ᶻᶻᶻ | SLEEP (HRS):

EXERCISE			IN A STATE OF KETOSIS?		
TYPE	TIME	DURATION	YES	NO	UNSURE

CRAVINGS			DAILY ENERGY LEVEL		
YES	NO	SOMEWHAT	HIGH	MEDIUM	LOW

MEALS

	BREAKFAST	
	FAT	GRAMS
	CARBS	GRAMS
	PROTEIN	GRAMS
	CALORIES	

	LUNCH	
	FAT	GRAMS
	CARBS	GRAMS
	PROTEIN	GRAMS
	CALORIES	

	DINNER	
	FAT	GRAMS
	CARBS	GRAMS
	PROTEIN	GRAMS
	CALORIES	

	SNACK	
	FAT	GRAMS
	CARBS	GRAMS
	PROTEIN	GRAMS
	CALORIES	

	SNACK	
	FAT	GRAMS
	CARBS	GRAMS
	PROTEIN	GRAMS
	CALORIES	

WATER INTAKE TRACKER

END OF THE DAY TOTAL OVERVIEW

CARBS	FAT	PROTEIN	CALORIES

DAILY TRACKER

DATE _____

SLEEP TRACKER:

RISE: _____   BEDTIME: _____   SLEEP (HRS): _____

EXERCISE			IN A STATE OF KETOSIS?		
TYPE	TIME	DURATION	YES	NO	UNSURE

CRAVINGS			DAILY ENERGY LEVEL		
YES	NO	SOMEWHAT	HIGH	MEDIUM	LOW

MEALS

BREAKFAST
FAT	GRAMS
CARBS	GRAMS
PROTEIN	GRAMS
CALORIES	

LUNCH
FAT	GRAMS
CARBS	GRAMS
PROTEIN	GRAMS
CALORIES	

DINNER
FAT	GRAMS
CARBS	GRAMS
PROTEIN	GRAMS
CALORIES	

SNACK
FAT	GRAMS
CARBS	GRAMS
PROTEIN	GRAMS
CALORIES	

SNACK
FAT	GRAMS
CARBS	GRAMS
PROTEIN	GRAMS
CALORIES	

WATER INTAKE TRACKER

END OF THE DAY TOTAL OVERVIEW

CARBS	FAT	PROTEIN	CALORIES

DAILY TRACKER

DATE _____

SLEEP TRACKER:

☀ RISE: _____   🌙 zᶻᶻ BEDTIME: _____   💭zᶻᶻ SLEEP (HRS): _____

EXERCISE			IN A STATE OF KETOSIS?		
TYPE	TIME	DURATION	YES	NO	UNSURE

CRAVINGS			DAILY ENERGY LEVEL		
YES	NO	SOMEWHAT	HIGH	MEDIUM	LOW

MEALS

	BREAKFAST	
	FAT	GRAMS
	CARBS	GRAMS
	PROTEIN	GRAMS
	CALORIES	

	LUNCH	
	FAT	GRAMS
	CARBS	GRAMS
	PROTEIN	GRAMS
	CALORIES	

	DINNER	
	FAT	GRAMS
	CARBS	GRAMS
	PROTEIN	GRAMS
	CALORIES	

	SNACK	
	FAT	GRAMS
	CARBS	GRAMS
	PROTEIN	GRAMS
	CALORIES	

	SNACK	
	FAT	GRAMS
	CARBS	GRAMS
	PROTEIN	GRAMS
	CALORIES	

WATER INTAKE TRACKER

💧 💧 💧 💧 💧 💧 💧 💧

END OF THE DAY TOTAL OVERVIEW

CARBS	FAT	PROTEIN	CALORIES

DAILY TRACKER

DATE _____

SLEEP TRACKER:

RISE: [   ]   BEDTIME: [   ]   SLEEP (HRS): [   ]

EXERCISE			IN A STATE OF KETOSIS?		
TYPE	TIME	DURATION	YES	NO	UNSURE

CRAVINGS			DAILY ENERGY LEVEL		
YES	NO	SOMEWHAT	HIGH	MEDIUM	LOW

MEALS

BREAKFAST
FAT	GRAMS
CARBS	GRAMS
PROTEIN	GRAMS
CALORIES	

LUNCH
FAT	GRAMS
CARBS	GRAMS
PROTEIN	GRAMS
CALORIES	

DINNER
FAT	GRAMS
CARBS	GRAMS
PROTEIN	GRAMS
CALORIES	

SNACK
FAT	GRAMS
CARBS	GRAMS
PROTEIN	GRAMS
CALORIES	

SNACK
FAT	GRAMS
CARBS	GRAMS
PROTEIN	GRAMS
CALORIES	

WATER INTAKE TRACKER

END OF THE DAY TOTAL OVERVIEW

CARBS	FAT	PROTEIN	CALORIES
[ ]	[ ]	[ ]	[ ]

DAILY TRACKER

DATE _____

SLEEP TRACKER:

☼ RISE: _____   🌙 zᶻz BEDTIME: _____   💭zᶻz SLEEP (HRS): _____

EXERCISE			IN A STATE OF KETOSIS?		
TYPE	TIME	DURATION	YES	NO	UNSURE

CRAVINGS			DAILY ENERGY LEVEL		
YES	NO	SOMEWHAT	HIGH	MEDIUM	LOW

MEALS

BREAKFAST
FAT .... GRAMS
CARBS .... GRAMS
PROTEIN .... GRAMS
CALORIES

LUNCH
FAT .... GRAMS
CARBS .... GRAMS
PROTEIN .... GRAMS
CALORIES

DINNER
FAT .... GRAMS
CARBS .... GRAMS
PROTEIN .... GRAMS
CALORIES

SNACK
FAT .... GRAMS
CARBS .... GRAMS
PROTEIN .... GRAMS
CALORIES

SNACK
FAT .... GRAMS
CARBS .... GRAMS
PROTEIN .... GRAMS
CALORIES

WATER INTAKE TRACKER

END OF THE DAY TOTAL OVERVIEW

CARBS	FAT	PROTEIN	CALORIES

DAILY TRACKER

DATE _____

SLEEP TRACKER:

RISE: _____   BEDTIME: _____   SLEEP (HRS): _____

EXERCISE			IN A STATE OF KETOSIS?		
TYPE	TIME	DURATION	YES	NO	UNSURE

CRAVINGS			DAILY ENERGY LEVEL		
YES	NO	SOMEWHAT	HIGH	MEDIUM	LOW

MEALS

	BREAKFAST	
	FAT	GRAMS
	CARBS	GRAMS
	PROTEIN	GRAMS
	CALORIES	

	LUNCH	
	FAT	GRAMS
	CARBS	GRAMS
	PROTEIN	GRAMS
	CALORIES	

	DINNER	
	FAT	GRAMS
	CARBS	GRAMS
	PROTEIN	GRAMS
	CALORIES	

	SNACK	
	FAT	GRAMS
	CARBS	GRAMS
	PROTEIN	GRAMS
	CALORIES	

	SNACK	
	FAT	GRAMS
	CARBS	GRAMS
	PROTEIN	GRAMS
	CALORIES	

WATER INTAKE TRACKER

END OF THE DAY TOTAL OVERVIEW

CARBS	FAT	PROTEIN	CALORIES

DAILY TRACKER

DATE _____

SLEEP TRACKER:

☀ RISE: _____   🌙 z$_z$^{z} BEDTIME: _____   💤 SLEEP (HRS): _____

EXERCISE			IN A STATE OF KETOSIS?		
TYPE	TIME	DURATION	YES	NO	UNSURE

CRAVINGS			DAILY ENERGY LEVEL		
YES	NO	SOMEWHAT	HIGH	MEDIUM	LOW

MEALS

		BREAKFAST
	FAT	GRAMS
	CARBS	GRAMS
	PROTEIN	GRAMS
	CALORIES	

		LUNCH
	FAT	GRAMS
	CARBS	GRAMS
	PROTEIN	GRAMS
	CALORIES	

		DINNER
	FAT	GRAMS
	CARBS	GRAMS
	PROTEIN	GRAMS
	CALORIES	

		SNACK
	FAT	GRAMS
	CARBS	GRAMS
	PROTEIN	GRAMS
	CALORIES	

		SNACK
	FAT	GRAMS
	CARBS	GRAMS
	PROTEIN	GRAMS
	CALORIES	

WATER INTAKE TRACKER

💧 💧 💧 💧 💧 💧 💧 💧

END OF THE DAY TOTAL OVERVIEW

CARBS	FAT	PROTEIN	CALORIES

DAILY TRACKER

DATE _____

SLEEP TRACKER:

☼ | RISE: | ☾ zᶻ | BEDTIME: | 💭zᶻ | SLEEP (HRS):

EXERCISE			IN A STATE OF KETOSIS?		
TYPE	TIME	DURATION	YES	NO	UNSURE

CRAVINGS			DAILY ENERGY LEVEL		
YES	NO	SOMEWHAT	HIGH	MEDIUM	LOW

MEALS

BREAKFAST
FAT	GRAMS
CARBS	GRAMS
PROTEIN	GRAMS
CALORIES	

LUNCH
FAT	GRAMS
CARBS	GRAMS
PROTEIN	GRAMS
CALORIES	

DINNER
FAT	GRAMS
CARBS	GRAMS
PROTEIN	GRAMS
CALORIES	

SNACK
FAT	GRAMS
CARBS	GRAMS
PROTEIN	GRAMS
CALORIES	

SNACK
FAT	GRAMS
CARBS	GRAMS
PROTEIN	GRAMS
CALORIES	

WATER INTAKE TRACKER

END OF THE DAY TOTAL OVERVIEW

CARBS	FAT	PROTEIN	CALORIES

DAILY TRACKER

DATE _____

SLEEP TRACKER:

☀ RISE: _____ 🌙 BEDTIME: _____ 💤 SLEEP (HRS): _____

EXERCISE			IN A STATE OF KETOSIS?		
TYPE	TIME	DURATION	YES	NO	UNSURE

CRAVINGS			DAILY ENERGY LEVEL		
YES	NO	SOMEWHAT	HIGH	MEDIUM	LOW

MEALS

	BREAKFAST	
	FAT	GRAMS
	CARBS	GRAMS
	PROTEIN	GRAMS
	CALORIES	

	LUNCH	
	FAT	GRAMS
	CARBS	GRAMS
	PROTEIN	GRAMS
	CALORIES	

	DINNER	
	FAT	GRAMS
	CARBS	GRAMS
	PROTEIN	GRAMS
	CALORIES	

	SNACK	
	FAT	GRAMS
	CARBS	GRAMS
	PROTEIN	GRAMS
	CALORIES	

	SNACK	
	FAT	GRAMS
	CARBS	GRAMS
	PROTEIN	GRAMS
	CALORIES	

WATER INTAKE TRACKER

END OF THE DAY TOTAL OVERVIEW

CARBS	FAT	PROTEIN	CALORIES

DAILY TRACKER

DATE _____

SLEEP TRACKER:

☀ RISE: _____   🌙 ᶻᶻᶻ BEDTIME: _____   💭ᶻᶻᶻ SLEEP (HRS): _____

EXERCISE			IN A STATE OF KETOSIS?		
TYPE	TIME	DURATION	YES	NO	UNSURE

CRAVINGS			DAILY ENERGY LEVEL		
YES	NO	SOMEWHAT	HIGH	MEDIUM	LOW

MEALS

BREAKFAST
FAT	GRAMS
CARBS	GRAMS
PROTEIN	GRAMS
CALORIES	

LUNCH
FAT	GRAMS
CARBS	GRAMS
PROTEIN	GRAMS
CALORIES	

DINNER
FAT	GRAMS
CARBS	GRAMS
PROTEIN	GRAMS
CALORIES	

SNACK
FAT	GRAMS
CARBS	GRAMS
PROTEIN	GRAMS
CALORIES	

SNACK
FAT	GRAMS
CARBS	GRAMS
PROTEIN	GRAMS
CALORIES	

WATER INTAKE TRACKER

END OF THE DAY TOTAL OVERVIEW

CARBS	FAT	PROTEIN	CALORIES

DAILY TRACKER

DATE _____

SLEEP TRACKER:

RISE: _____ BEDTIME: _____ SLEEP (HRS): _____

EXERCISE			IN A STATE OF KETOSIS?		
TYPE	TIME	DURATION	YES	NO	UNSURE

CRAVINGS			DAILY ENERGY LEVEL		
YES	NO	SOMEWHAT	HIGH	MEDIUM	LOW

MEALS

BREAKFAST
FAT		GRAMS
CARBS		GRAMS
PROTEIN		GRAMS
CALORIES		

LUNCH
FAT		GRAMS
CARBS		GRAMS
PROTEIN		GRAMS
CALORIES		

DINNER
FAT		GRAMS
CARBS		GRAMS
PROTEIN		GRAMS
CALORIES		

SNACK
FAT		GRAMS
CARBS		GRAMS
PROTEIN		GRAMS
CALORIES		

SNACK
FAT		GRAMS
CARBS		GRAMS
PROTEIN		GRAMS
CALORIES		

WATER INTAKE TRACKER

END OF THE DAY TOTAL OVERVIEW

CARBS	FAT	PROTEIN	CALORIES

DAILY TRACKER

DATE _____

SLEEP TRACKER:

☀ RISE: _____   🌙 BEDTIME: _____   💤 SLEEP (HRS): _____

EXERCISE			IN A STATE OF KETOSIS?		
TYPE	TIME	DURATION	YES	NO	UNSURE

CRAVINGS			DAILY ENERGY LEVEL		
YES	NO	SOMEWHAT	HIGH	MEDIUM	LOW

MEALS

	BREAKFAST	
	FAT	GRAMS
	CARBS	GRAMS
	PROTEIN	GRAMS
	CALORIES	

	LUNCH	
	FAT	GRAMS
	CARBS	GRAMS
	PROTEIN	GRAMS
	CALORIES	

	DINNER	
	FAT	GRAMS
	CARBS	GRAMS
	PROTEIN	GRAMS
	CALORIES	

	SNACK	
	FAT	GRAMS
	CARBS	GRAMS
	PROTEIN	GRAMS
	CALORIES	

	SNACK	
	FAT	GRAMS
	CARBS	GRAMS
	PROTEIN	GRAMS
	CALORIES	

WATER INTAKE TRACKER

END OF THE DAY TOTAL OVERVIEW

CARBS	FAT	PROTEIN	CALORIES

DAILY TRACKER

DATE _____

SLEEP TRACKER:

☀ RISE: _____   🌙 zzz BEDTIME: _____   💤 SLEEP (HRS): _____

EXERCISE			IN A STATE OF KETOSIS?		
TYPE	TIME	DURATION	YES	NO	UNSURE

CRAVINGS			DAILY ENERGY LEVEL		
YES	NO	SOMEWHAT	HIGH	MEDIUM	LOW

MEALS

	BREAKFAST	
	FAT	GRAMS
	CARBS	GRAMS
	PROTEIN	GRAMS
	CALORIES	

	LUNCH	
	FAT	GRAMS
	CARBS	GRAMS
	PROTEIN	GRAMS
	CALORIES	

	DINNER	
	FAT	GRAMS
	CARBS	GRAMS
	PROTEIN	GRAMS
	CALORIES	

	SNACK	
	FAT	GRAMS
	CARBS	GRAMS
	PROTEIN	GRAMS
	CALORIES	

	SNACK	
	FAT	GRAMS
	CARBS	GRAMS
	PROTEIN	GRAMS
	CALORIES	

WATER INTAKE TRACKER

END OF THE DAY TOTAL OVERVIEW

CARBS	FAT	PROTEIN	CALORIES

INTERMITTENT FASTING

DATES:

	START TIME	END TIME	TOTAL HOURS
MON			
TUE	:	:	
WED	:	:	
THU	;	;	
FRI	:	:	
SAT	:	:	
SUN	:	:	

DATES:

	START TIME	END TIME	TOTAL HOURS
MON			
TUE	:	:	
WED	:	:	
THU	;	;	
FRI	:	:	
SAT	:	:	
SUN	:	:	

DATES:

	START TIME	END TIME	TOTAL HOURS
MON			
TUE	:	:	
WED	:	:	
THU	;	;	
FRI	:	:	
SAT	:	:	
SUN	:	:	

DATES:

	START TIME	END TIME	TOTAL HOURS
MON			
TUE	:	:	
WED	:	:	
THU	;	;	
FRI	:	:	
SAT	:	:	
SUN	:	:	

DATES:

	START TIME	END TIME	TOTAL HOURS
MON			
TUE	:	:	
WED	:	:	
THU	;	;	
FRI	:	:	
SAT	:	:	
SUN	:	:	

DATES:

	START TIME	END TIME	TOTAL HOURS
MON			
TUE	:	:	
WED	:	:	
THU	;	;	
FRI	:	:	
SAT	:	:	
SUN	:	:	

DATES:

	START TIME	END TIME	TOTAL HOURS
MON			
TUE	:	:	
WED	:	:	
THU	;	;	
FRI	:	:	
SAT	:	:	
SUN	:	:	

DATES:

	START TIME	END TIME	TOTAL HOURS
MON			
TUE	:	:	
WED	:	:	
THU	;	;	
FRI	:	:	
SAT	:	:	
SUN	:	:	

DATES:

	START TIME	END TIME	TOTAL HOURS
MON			
TUE	:	:	
WED	:	:	
THU	;	;	
FRI	:	:	
SAT	:	:	
SUN	:	:	

NOTES

INTERMITTENT FASTING

DATES:			
	START TIME	END TIME	TOTAL HOURS
MON			
TUE	:	:	
WED	:	:	
THU	;	;	
FRI	:	:	
SAT	:	:	
SUN	:	:	

DATES:			
	START TIME	END TIME	TOTAL HOURS
MON			
TUE	:	:	
WED	:	:	
THU	;	;	
FRI	:	:	
SAT	:	:	
SUN	:	:	

DATES:			
	START TIME	END TIME	TOTAL HOURS
MON			
TUE	:	:	
WED	:	:	
THU	;	;	
FRI	:	:	
SAT	:	:	
SUN	:	:	

DATES:			
	START TIME	END TIME	TOTAL HOURS
MON			
TUE	:	:	
WED	:	:	
THU	;	;	
FRI	:	:	
SAT	:	:	
SUN	:	:	

DATES:			
	START TIME	END TIME	TOTAL HOURS
MON			
TUE	:	:	
WED	:	:	
THU	;	;	
FRI	:	:	
SAT	:	:	
SUN	:	:	

DATES:			
	START TIME	END TIME	TOTAL HOURS
MON			
TUE	:	:	
WED	:	:	
THU	;	;	
FRI	:	:	
SAT	:	:	
SUN	:	:	

DATES:			
	START TIME	END TIME	TOTAL HOURS
MON			
TUE	:	:	
WED	:	:	
THU	;	;	
FRI	:	:	
SAT	:	:	
SUN	:	:	

DATES:			
	START TIME	END TIME	TOTAL HOURS
MON			
TUE	:	:	
WED	:	:	
THU	;	;	
FRI	:	:	
SAT	:	:	
SUN	:	:	

DATES:			
	START TIME	END TIME	TOTAL HOURS
MON			
TUE	:	:	
WED	:	:	
THU	;	;	
FRI	:	:	
SAT	:	:	
SUN	:	:	

NOTES

90 DAYS OF KETO

STARTING WEIGHT:

DAY 90 WEIGHT:

1	2	3	4	5	6	7	8	9	10	LBS LOST: INCHES LOST:
11	12	13	14	15	16	17	18	19	20	LBS LOST: INCHES LOST:
21	22	23	24	25	26	27	28	29	30	LBS LOST: INCHES LOST:
31	32	33	34	35	36	37	38	39	40	LBS LOST: INCHES LOST:
41	42	43	44	45	46	47	48	49	50	LBS LOST: INCHES LOST:
51	52	53	54	55	56	57	58	59	60	LBS LOST: INCHES LOST:
61	62	63	64	65	66	67	68	69	70	LBS LOST: INCHES LOST:
71	72	73	74	75	76	77	78	79	80	LBS LOST: INCHES LOST:
81	82	83	84	85	86	87	88	89	90	LBS LOST: INCHES LOST:

TOTAL WEIGHT LOST:

TOTAL INCHES LOST:

THOUGHTS & REFLECTIONS:

KETO RECIPES

RECIPE FOR:

AMOUNT	INGREDIENTS

DIRECTIONS

NOTES

SERVES	
PREP TIME	
COOK TIME	
TOOLS	
TEMP	

CARBS	
FAT	
PROTEIN	
CALORIES	

KETO RECIPES

RECIPE FOR:

AMOUNT	INGREDIENTS

DIRECTIONS

NOTES

SERVES	
PREP TIME	
COOK TIME	
TOOLS	
TEMP	

CARBS	
FAT	
PROTEIN	
CALORIES	

KETO RECIPES

RECIPE FOR:

AMOUNT	INGREDIENTS

DIRECTIONS

NOTES

SERVES	
PREP TIME	
COOK TIME	
TOOLS	
TEMP	

CARBS	
FAT	
PROTEIN	
CALORIES	

KETO RECIPES

RECIPE FOR:

AMOUNT	INGREDIENTS

DIRECTIONS

NOTES

SERVES	
PREP TIME	
COOK TIME	
TOOLS	
TEMP	

CARBS	
FAT	
PROTEIN	
CALORIES	

KETO RECIPES

RECIPE FOR:

AMOUNT	INGREDIENTS	DIRECTIONS

NOTES

SERVES	
PREP TIME	
COOK TIME	
TOOLS	
TEMP	

CARBS	
FAT	
PROTEIN	
CALORIES	

KETO RECIPES

RECIPE FOR:

AMOUNT	INGREDIENTS

DIRECTIONS

NOTES

SERVES	
PREP TIME	
COOK TIME	
TOOLS	
TEMP	

CARBS	
FAT	
PROTEIN	
CALORIES	

KETO RECIPES

RECIPE FOR:

AMOUNT	INGREDIENTS	DIRECTIONS

NOTES			
	SERVES	
	PREP TIME	
	COOK TIME	
	TOOLS	
	TEMP	
	CARBS	
	FAT	
	PROTEIN	
	CALORIES	

KETO RECIPES

RECIPE FOR:

AMOUNT	INGREDIENTS

DIRECTIONS

NOTES

SERVES	
PREP TIME	
COOK TIME	
TOOLS	
TEMP	

CARBS	
FAT	
PROTEIN	
CALORIES	

KETO RECIPES

RECIPE FOR:

AMOUNT	INGREDIENTS	DIRECTIONS

NOTES		

SERVES	
PREP TIME	
COOK TIME	
TOOLS	
TEMP	

CARBS	
FAT	
PROTEIN	
CALORIES	

KETO RECIPES

RECIPE FOR:

AMOUNT	INGREDIENTS	DIRECTIONS

NOTES		
	SERVES	
	PREP TIME	
	COOK TIME	
	TOOLS	
	TEMP	
	CARBS	
	FAT	
	PROTEIN	
	CALORIES	

KETO RECIPES

RECIPE FOR:

AMOUNT	INGREDIENTS

DIRECTIONS

NOTES

SERVES	
PREP TIME	
COOK TIME	
TOOLS	
TEMP	

CARBS	
FAT	
PROTEIN	
CALORIES	

KETO RECIPES

RECIPE FOR:

AMOUNT	INGREDIENTS	DIRECTIONS

NOTES

SERVES	
PREP TIME	
COOK TIME	
TOOLS	
TEMP	

CARBS	
FAT	
PROTEIN	
CALORIES	

KETO RECIPES

RECIPE FOR:

AMOUNT	INGREDIENTS	DIRECTIONS

NOTES

SERVES	
PREP TIME	
COOK TIME	
TOOLS	
TEMP	

CARBS	
FAT	
PROTEIN	
CALORIES	

KETO RECIPES

RECIPE FOR:

AMOUNT	INGREDIENTS

DIRECTIONS

NOTES

SERVES	
PREP TIME	
COOK TIME	
TOOLS	
TEMP	

CARBS	
FAT	
PROTEIN	
CALORIES	

KETO RECIPES

RECIPE FOR:

AMOUNT	INGREDIENTS

DIRECTIONS

NOTES

SERVES	
PREP TIME	
COOK TIME	
TOOLS	
TEMP	

CARBS	
FAT	
PROTEIN	
CALORIES	

KETO RECIPES

RECIPE FOR:

AMOUNT	INGREDIENTS	DIRECTIONS

NOTES		
	SERVES	
	PREP TIME	
	COOK TIME	
	TOOLS	
	TEMP	
	CARBS	
	FAT	
	PROTEIN	
	CALORIES	

KETO RECIPES

RECIPE FOR:

AMOUNT	INGREDIENTS

DIRECTIONS

NOTES

SERVES	
PREP TIME	
COOK TIME	
TOOLS	
TEMP	

CARBS	
FAT	
PROTEIN	
CALORIES	

KETO RECIPES

RECIPE FOR:

AMOUNT	INGREDIENTS	DIRECTIONS

NOTES

SERVES	
PREP TIME	
COOK TIME	
TOOLS	
TEMP	

CARBS	
FAT	
PROTEIN	
CALORIES	

KETO RECIPES

RECIPE FOR:

AMOUNT	INGREDIENTS

DIRECTIONS

NOTES

SERVES	
PREP TIME	
COOK TIME	
TOOLS	
TEMP	

CARBS	
FAT	
PROTEIN	
CALORIES	

KETO RECIPES

RECIPE FOR:

AMOUNT	INGREDIENTS	DIRECTIONS

NOTES		
	SERVES	
	PREP TIME	
	COOK TIME	
	TOOLS	
	TEMP	
	CARBS	
	FAT	
	PROTEIN	
	CALORIES	

KETO RECIPES

RECIPE FOR:

AMOUNT	INGREDIENTS	DIRECTIONS

NOTES		
	SERVES	
	PREP TIME	
	COOK TIME	
	TOOLS	
	TEMP	
	CARBS	
	FAT	
	PROTEIN	
	CALORIES	

www.ingramcontent.com/pod-product-compliance
Lightning Source LLC
Chambersburg PA
CBHW052113020426
42335CB00021B/2747